More Advance Praise for *Beat Breast Cancer Like a Boss*

"If there were a bible of boss women who beat breast cancer, *Beat Breast Cancer Like a Boss* would be it. Sheryl Crow, Edie Falco, and Jill Kargman, among other powerhouses, offer their true testaments on how to survive cancer to inspire any woman to be the CEO of her comeback."

> —Marisa Acocella, *New York Times* Bestselling Author of *Ann Tenna* and *Cancer Vixen*

"Filled with raw stories of hope, resilience, and strength, *Beat Breast Cancer Like a Boss* is an essential companion for those living with and being treated for breast cancer. Although progress continues to be made in the fight against breast cancer, this disease still strikes one in eight American women. *Beat Breast Cancer Like a Boss* documents the challenges of a breast cancer diagnosis and treatment, while encouraging readers to be their own advocates and, ultimately, beat cancer like a boss."

> —Claudine Isaacs, M.D., Associate Director for Clinical Research and Leader Clinical Breast Cancer Program at Georgetown Lombardi Comprehensive Cancer Center

"This book is the most comprehensive guide to all sorts of questions the doctors can't answer and the most original advice I've read on how to deal with any uncertain and daunting situation. Buy this book for anyone going through breast cancer treatment, any survivor, and any woman at risk who might be scared. *Beat Breast Cancer Like a Boss* isn't just for women touched by cancer—it is a manual for how to survive any curve ball in life."

> —Geralyn Lucas, Author of *Why I Wore Lipstick To My Mastectomy* and *Then Came Life*

For more information, email info@diversionbooks.com

Diversion Books
A division of Diversion Publishing Corp.
www.diversionbooks.com

First Diversion Books edition, September 2020
Paperback ISBN: 978-1-63576-713-1
eBook ISBN: 978-1-63576-710-0

Printed in The United States of America

1 3 5 7 9 10 8 6 4 2

Library of Congress cataloging-in-publication data is available on file.

If you picked up this book because you are,
or someone you love is, going through a difficult time,
this book is for you.

CONTENTS

PREFACE

TODAY, I AM a seasoned TV producer and reporter with ten years of covering the White House, State Department, and Capitol Hill under my belt. I've been in plenty of high-stakes situations where it pays to be cool, calm, and collected, whether it's writing a scoop on deadline, chasing senators through the basement of the Capitol building, or grilling the White House press secretary in the briefing room.

But ten years ago, I was a scared-out-of-my-mind college senior who had just found out I had a genetic mutation that made it likely—about 80 percent likely—that I would probably develop breast cancer at some point. The memory is crystal clear in my mind, down to the fact that my mom and I got a bit day-drunk on Sauvignon Blanc before we sat down with the genetic counselor to get the test results. A few weeks earlier, I had gone over my family history with the counselor. I watched as she marked down all the women on my dad's side of the family tree that had been diagnosed with breast and ovarian cancer, representing them with scary little black triangles. I had been an excellent candidate for BRCA testing, and then my blood test results came back positive. I had always prided myself on acing tests. Not this one.

I was in a panic and had no idea where to turn. I was just a college kid—I wasn't supposed to be thinking about breast cancer! Besides a few words about having my own children before age thirty-five, my genetic counselor didn't give me a lot of advice. So I met with a few doctors, one of whom told me she was seeing more and more young women opt for a prophylactic bilateral mastectomy and reconstructive surgery.

It didn't take long for me to realize that that was the right choice for me. I no longer viewed my breasts as assets; they were ticking time bombs. Plus, they were a little small. So I looked on the bright side and viewed the procedures as a win-win: Defuse the bomb on my chest, and get an ancillary upgrade! I also knew that my family had the resources to pay for whatever insurance did not cover, which ended up being quite a bit.

But I also had all sorts of questions that the doctors couldn't really answer. What was the best time in my life to take two weeks off to have life-changing surgery? Should I do it while in college, or should I wait until I was out in the "real world"? Would I miss my natural breasts? What about dating? When was the right time to disclose to potential boyfriends that I was in various stages of chest renovation? And when I did decide to have the surgery in college, I got so many questions about why I was doing this at such a young age. Didn't I want to keep my breasts until I snagged a husband? What about losing out on the joys of breastfeeding? My favorite inquisitor was the nurse who, as she prepped me for my implant surgery, asked me if I wasn't too young to be having this procedure. Jig's up, ma'am.

So overall, I was lucky. I went through that whole period quite bravely and defiantly. Besides those initial few days of panic, I never looked back and ended up answering many of those questions myself. (Have the surgery while in college before you have to miss time at work; you won't miss your natural breasts; no guy worth a second date will have an issue with this.) Nevertheless, I often felt as though I was traveling this road alone.

My mastectomy took place several years before women like Angelina Jolie and Christina Applegate went public with their experiences, putting beautiful, famous faces on the BRCA gene and making it much easier for me to explain what I had. But their stories did more for me than provide a shorthand description of my affliction ("I have the Angelina Jolie gene"); even years after my surgeries, I felt a sense of camaraderie with these famous women. They went through what I did! They felt the same things I felt! Maybe they asked themselves the same questions I had, too.

My experience has led me to appreciate that when you're going through a trial, community matters. That's why I decided to write this book. It helps to hear from and connect with other people who have been through similar experiences—not just to seek advice, but also simply to commiserate. I've also come to understand that connecting with well-known people, even if it's just reading something in their voice, can help people understand that they are not alone. That was my experience when I first read Angelina Jolie's story. We can't all call up our favorite celebrity or professional hero with breast cancer to talk about what it was like for her (or him), but I wrote this book in an attempt to provide the next best thing.

It's true that the women whose stories grace the pages of this book have almost all reached some level of professional success that has given them access and resources that, unfortunately, are not available to many women in the United States and, indeed, the world. Regardless, there are many other aspects of breast cancer that have no correlation to fame or resources. Frankly, I was surprised to learn how even these incredibly savvy women could face the same challenges in an exam room that any of us might: not having their concerns be taken seriously by a doctor; getting medical advice and then debating going against it; grappling with disruptions to family life.

Also, I made a concerted effort to represent a broad spectrum of breast cancer stories from women of different ages and ethnic backgrounds. These include everyone from a twenty-three-year-old white ballerina diagnosed with stage IV metastatic breast cancer, to an Asian American financial executive living overseas, to a powerful African American state attorney general who battled the disease—and won—three times.

My hope in writing this book is that, even if you've never had to sneak into a hospital to avoid paparazzi, you can relate to aspects of each woman's breast cancer battle. And that reading about those aspects will help you get through your own experience, whether you're fighting the disease yourself, taking care of someone who is, or you just want to be a good support system for someone you care about.

This book has been a labor of love, written in the early mornings and late nights (and the occasional slow news day at work). The stories of these incredible women have brought me to tears several times through the course of putting it together. It doesn't matter where you are in life, what stage of breast cancer (or any cancer, frankly!) you have, or how far along you are in your journey. I know that if you've picked up this book, you're going to find inspiration in these delightfully varied, yet universally resonant, stories of struggle and resilience against one of the greatest health challenges women face today.

INTRODUCTION
COKIE'S STORY

COKIE ROBERTS WAS a trailblazing journalist and author, a co-anchor of *This Week*, the ABC Sunday news show, from 1996 to 2002, and a reporter for NPR. I was blessed to call her a colleague while I was a producer at ABC News. And, like so many other young, female journalists, I was the beneficiary of her expertise and sage insight. Every once in a while she'd send me a quick note, responding to some email I had sent with Capitol Hill editorial guidance. I had grown up watching and admiring Cokie, so I got a rush every time I saw her name in my inbox, relishing her emails which always contained a quick word of support or advice. You'd be surprised to learn how many of the women whose reporting you read, watch, or listen to have at some point spent time under Cokie's wing.

Cokie was also a proud breast cancer survivor and fierce advocate for funding for research and access to treatment, especially for low-income women. She took up the cause well before she herself was diagnosed in 2002, and she faced that trial with humor, optimism, and courage.

Here's Cokie in her own words.

I got the diagnosis [in 2002] and then I went to the beach. And then when I came back I started dealing with it. It's not like it was going to grow to my liver while I was at the beach! I was just gone a couple weeks.

I wasn't terrified because I knew enough about it, and I knew it wasn't a death sentence. I knew it was going to be a big fat pain and that it was not going to be something I was going to enjoy, but I was not in this state of just horror that I think a lot of people are.

Cokie had a supernatural ability to keep things in perspective, in part because she'd already lived through several family tragedies. When she was twenty-eight, her father, House Majority Leader Hale Boggs, perished in a plane crash. In 1990, Cokie's sister Barbara died of ocular melanoma. Cokie had also started advocating for breast cancer research years before her own bout.

> The next year [after Barbara died], two friends of mine died of breast cancer, and they were in adjoining rooms at the funeral home. The masses were staggered so everybody could go to both. And I just got mad. I wrote an op-ed for the *Washington Post* that was picked up around the country. At that point, the funding for all of cancer and all of heart disease combined was less than the funding for AIDS. And of course, I'm for AIDS funding, but that was because of advocacy.
>
> I do remember doing *Nightline* one night where I was the anchor, and there was some new data out on breast cancer. I insisted on doing a whole show on it, and they basically treated me like I wasn't there, like I was just invisible. And everybody was just eye-rolling.
>
> I remember saying to the executive producer, "You know, men really might care because they want someone to fold their socks." And, of course, it turned out to be an incredibly well-watched show because it affects so many people.
>
> This was before I got breast cancer. There was no breast cancer in the family; there was no reason to think I would be a beneficiary of my own activities. And then I was diagnosed.

Cokie's breast cancer was lobular, meaning it did not form into lumps like the sort of breast cancer that forms in a woman's milk ducts. Instead it was diffuse, spreading itself out within the breast tissue in a line formation. That makes it harder to detect, but Cokie's attentive OB-GYN noticed a hardening in her breast, even before she had a mammogram.

I then had a mammogram, and it was not all that definitive. And so then you start the sonograms and MRIs and all that. And then they did a biopsy, and it was positive. I had had a biopsy before, years before, and it had been negative, so I was not necessarily primed for it being positive, but I was not surprised.

I immediately had a lumpectomy, to the degree that you can excise lobular cancer. And with it a sentinel node dissection. My doctor had said, "I'd be amazed if there's node involvement." And then they pulled out the sentinel node and it was cancerous, and nine of thirteen nodes were cancerous. So that was the moment of truth. Because up until that point, I thought, "I can get away with radiation."

Once I got the diagnosis about the nodes, I was frightened. But then we started on a course of chemotherapy and radiation, and then it was just putting one foot in front of the other.

[When I realized I would have to have chemo], I also realized that I would have to go public. Because I was going to lose my hair and all that, and I was still anchoring *This Week*. And the hardest part about that was telling my mother, because my sister had died of cancer. I was very distressed about it. I just didn't want her to have to go through [what she did with Barbara].

Cokie's mother, Rep. Lindy Boggs, had been elected to her late husband's seat and served in Congress for seventeen years. She also served as U.S. ambassador to the Vatican. Lindy died in 2013.

My brother and sister-in-law and my husband and I set up a dinner. We were in a private room in a restaurant, and I told her then. But my mother was tough. She had been through a lot, and she handled it fine.

Cokie also had to break the news to the rest of her family: her husband, Steve, and their two adult children.

I told my husband, and I told him I didn't want to tell anybody, which is my MO. And then he sounded all glum, talking to the children, and they kept saying, "What's wrong?" And he said, "You have to talk to your mother." So, without betraying my trust, he outed me anyway, right? And so I then told them, and everybody just moved on from there.

The next step in Cokie's disclosure gauntlet was telling her colleagues at ABC.

I had already said to all of my bosses, before I was diagnosed with breast cancer, that I was not going to renew my contract. So they all knew that. But then when the cancer diagnosis came, I wanted to make it clear that it had nothing to do with my decision to leave the show.

But somebody from the hospital called the *Washington Post*, so we couldn't really manage it entirely the way we wanted to. And at that point, Lloyd Grove was writing the gossip column, so I talked to him, and he was very respectful. Basically his reaction was, "You get to handle this the way you want." There were two things I didn't want people to think: I didn't want them to think that I had been, in any way, duplicitous when I made the announcement about leaving the show. I didn't want them to think that I really had something else that I was not telling them. But the other thing was that I didn't want breast cancer [sufferers] to think that you had to quit your job!

Now that her news was out, though, Cokie had to deal with other people's reactions to it, which proved alternately heartening and exhausting.

I remember when my father's plane went down, and people just didn't know what to say. They'd cross the street rather than talk to you. But by and large people couldn't have been nicer and more supportive. I got thousands of letters, and that was very comforting in one way, but it was also a burden, because I needed to answer them.

It was total strangers who knew everything about you. That was sort of weird. And having someone come up to you in the airport and say, "I'm praying for you," just seemed kind of an invasion of privacy. But then my reaction was, "You jerk—really—these are people who are caring about you and kind and considerate in every way." And I did come to see it as sort of a cushion of support.

Cokie was lucky to have friends and family accompany her to the chemo sessions, and her radiation schedule was convenient.

Anytime I had chemo, a friend took me, and that meant sitting in the hospital with me for eight hours. And I was asleep for part of it and awake for part of it. But in the crazy busy life we lead, it was a nice time to just be alone with friends that you never get time with! It turned out to have some very positive aspects.

Then with radiation, which is daily, they were great about setting it at 7 in the morning so I could just dash on over and have the radiation and then have my whole day. That was a piece of cake.

But she also had to deal with losing her hair in a very public way.

I hated the wigs. It's so funny because a lot of people wear wigs all the time. And I was surprised to hate it so much because I have horrible hair and I've always had horrible hair, and I thought, "Well that will be a cinch." And I actually have a nice-looking head. I didn't mind myself looking at myself bald. But other people did, and there was no getting comfortable.

Even after she was diagnosed, Cokie remained more concerned about other people's well-being. Once breast cancer awareness became a fully realized cause, and consumers could show their support by buying anything pink, she began focusing on advocating for equality of care—particularly for low-income women in Washington, D.C., which has one of the highest breast cancer rates in the world.

Our whole health care system is horrible, but when you're doing advocacy now, it's still very important to raise the funds for research, because it's making a big difference.

Where the gap is—and it's an enormous gap—is in the delivery of services, particularly in underserved neighborhoods. And so here in the District of Columbia, it's one of the highest mortality rates for breast cancer in the world, which is shocking and appalling.

I think it's very important that people understand that this is not a disease that has been conquered, even though great strides have been made. And there's still a lot of work to do, particularly in terms of getting people treatment who need the treatment.

As a life-long journalist, being a voice for others came naturally to Cokie. It was using her voice to talk about herself that was hard. She was always so focused on being the provider of help, the source of confidence, the shoulder to cry on.

> People are just distressed for you. And they want you to be OK and they feel really sad that you're not. And so I think it's very common to just say, "Don't worry about it. I'll be OK."
>
> The hardest part for me by far was accepting help. You know, I'm always the person who helps everybody else. And people really wanted to be helpful, and I had to understand that it was a gift they were giving me, but it was also a gift for me to say yes.
>
> And so that was hard, but I did it, and I'm very glad that I did it.

Here's what I didn't know when I recorded this interview on August 9, 2017: Cokie had found out her cancer came back the previous summer, fourteen years later. It had metastasized to other parts of her body. She and her husband Steve were informed that this cancer was aggressive.

For the interview, Cokie and I sat down together in her office, which was on the same floor as mine. She had known for at least a year that her cancer had returned, but she graciously answered forty minutes of questions about her advocacy work, her diagnosis, and her 2002 battle. She never mentioned—never even alluded to—the fact that she was actively in the fight again. But I think that was her goal. Cokie never let cancer get in the way of her living her life on her terms. She was defiantly focused on the things that matter most: friends, a career she loved, and helping lift up the people around her, like me.

Frankly, during our interview, I probably didn't have as good an understanding, as I do now, that beating breast cancer comes in different forms. There I was, asking her about what it was like to "beat" this disease, as if it had come and gone, to be relegated permanently to her rearview mirror. I didn't realize at the time that she existed in the state of beating breast cancer from her first diagnosis until the day she died.

The title of this book is *Beat Breast Cancer Like A Boss*, and it contains stories and tips to help you do just that. But it's essential that you know that there is no one definition of the word "beat" in this context. It's not a win-or-lose proposition. Everyone "beats" cancer in their own way.

The most standard interpretation, I suppose, would be what you think it would be: to complete treatment for breast cancer (or any other cancer), go into remission, and remain cancer-free for the rest of your life. That's certainly one way.

But another way to beat cancer is to not let it prevent you from being you, no matter what stage of treatment or recovery you're in. To keep living your life, even if you have to make some changes. To pursue your passions, even if that takes on a different shape than you thought it might. To spend time with the people you love, even if your relationships evolve, because sometimes cancer can do that. Many of the women in this book beat—and are continuing to beat—breast cancer in this way.

But no one embodies it more than the late Cokie Roberts.

Cokie, I think you knew, when we had our interview, that you were teaching me a lesson I wouldn't learn right away. I've learned it now. Thank you.

PART I

THE
CREATIVES

THE WOMEN PROFILED in this section are all driven by a desire to create and express themselves through art, whether it's music, dance, drama, literature, or architecture. But when diagnosed with breast cancer, each used her creative outlets differently.

Some turned their battle into art. The supporting character in one of Barbara Delinsky's novels, a breast cancer survivor, ended up inspiring so many readers that it motivated Delinsky to create a nonfiction compilation of stories from other survivors.

Others used art as a source of stability and consistency when their lives were unexpectedly plunged into chaos. Actress Edie Falco was able to put cancer on pause when she stepped in front of the camera. Maggie Kudirka, the "Bald Ballerina," defied her doctor's orders by returning to the barre days after surgery, because it was essential for her mental health.

Still others had to turn off the creative spigot entirely, choosing to return to it only when they were on the other side of cancer. Singer Sheryl Crow didn't open her songwriting notebook from her diagnosis until she was cancer-free, recognizing that in order to fully awaken herself to the experience of breast cancer, she had to dispose of the creative screen she often hid behind.

Each had her own reason for either diving deeper into creative expression or setting it aside entirely. But in the end, breast cancer had an indelible effect on their art, just as it did on their lives.

SHERYL CROW

You realize, "Oh, wait a minute. I thought I was controlling everything, but I'm actually not controlling everything. I actually don't have control over anything." And I think it's terribly scary and daunting and then it becomes liberating.

■ ■ ■

Sheryl Crow is a multi-Grammy-winning singer-songwriter, with such hits as "If It Makes You Happy," "Soak Up the Sun," "All I Wanna Do," and "Everyday is a Winding Road." Her most recent album, *Threads*, was released in August 2019 and features collaborations with her favorite artists and close friends.

When Sheryl Crow performs, it looks, sounds, and feels effortless—as if she landed on the stage out of nowhere and someone handed her a guitar. As if, five minutes before, she was hanging out with friends and just decided to have some fun and sing some of her hit songs.

In reality, Sheryl's orchestrating a churning machine of people, schedules, logistics, and obligations, all the while trying to find enough space in her mind and in the day to keep growing and creating as an artist. Of course, she has a professional football-sized team of people whose job it is to take care of her, but in turn, it's her job to take care of all of them. Without Sheryl Crow the person, there is no Sheryl Crow the tour, the album, the brand. It all falls apart.

That's a lot of pressure. Even if, like Sheryl Crow, you make it look effortless.

I've always shown up for everything that was expected of me. I've always delivered on everything.

It was only after she was diagnosed with breast cancer that she decided, for the first time in her adult life, to show up for herself before anyone else.

THE DIAGNOSIS

When she was diagnosed at age forty-four, Crow was the embodiment of health. She worked out religiously, she ate healthfully, and she had no family history of cancer.

My OB-GYN started me with doing mammograms at age thirty-five because I had had several cyst-like masses—I had several lumps that were suspect and required needle biopsies. And then once I hit forty, I went every year. I was a picture of good health. Very fit. Ate well, no family history. Not the typical candidate for breast cancer. And yet, I fell into that statistic of one in eight women who winds up being diagnosed.

I had a mammogram that looked suspect and my OB-GYN said, "Look, let's not wait the six months. Let's just go ahead and see what's going on." And it turned out to be invasive. Her mom was going through breast cancer treatment and had been one of those who waited six months. She felt it was imperative for whoever's told "wait six months" to go ahead do their due diligence. So I had a needle biopsy in both breasts and had a lumpectomy done in both breasts. And I was invasive in one and not in the other.

Sheryl had two factors working against her, which thankfully didn't stop her doctor from her due diligence. She had dense breasts, which were much harder to screen when she was diagnosed (the technology has improved since then). Plus, she was a relatively young woman.

["Dense breasts"] isn't a phrase that every woman hears, even when they have dense breasts. And when you do hear it doesn't mean you know what it means. With technology changing and with there being 3D technology for screening, we're able to see so much more clearly, fewer false positives, less "come back in six months."

I hear these crazy horror stories every day about younger women who sense that there's something going on. And they aren't being taken seriously. And they're misdiagnosed. We should take women seriously when they say they feel like something is going on. It's daunting and it's also a colossal hassle to go from one doctor to another to be taken seriously. At a certain point when enough doctors say there's nothing wrong with you, you have to believe that.

Sheryl was also going through a very public breakup with her ex-fiancé, Lance Armstrong, when she learned she had breast cancer.

[The diagnosis] was a much bigger blow than probably it would have been had I not been alone in it. And there is something to that feeling of aloneness when you're diagnosed with breast cancer anyway, because the reality I find is that there's a connection to breast cancer with being a woman in general, and not just because of the physical breast, but because of what it represents. We are caretakers by nature. And I think oftentimes, we're used to taking care of everyone but ourselves.

So being newly out of a relationship and having my so-called life partner not be there and to realize that, "Wait a minute—he couldn't fix that anyway. I've been taking care of him and not taking care of me." It was a real stand-up moment for me. I had to learn how to voice my needs, to voice my wants and desires, and to be brutally honest with those around me, and I also had to learn how to let people take care of me.

I remember exactly how I felt and the look on my surgical oncologist's face [when she revealed my diagnosis]. Those memories are as fresh as they were the minute they happened. And I remember where I was at in my life—my life was sort of at a moment of tumult. And so it was just an imposition to even be in the middle of having to deal with needle biopsies and lumpectomies, when I felt like my personal life was sort of on the skids. And I appreciated the fact that the woman who gave me the news was also the woman that walked through the experience with me. We've maintained a very strong friendship ever since.

THE BATTLE

Putting her "caretaker" role to the side was not only essential to Sheryl's recovery; it also allowed her to make more meaningful connections with others.

My radiologist said something interesting, "Don't miss out on the cancer lesson. I can't tell you what it is, but don't miss out on it." I've had so many women come up to me and tell their breast cancer story. And almost without exception, the story is, "I had to learn how to put myself first. I had to learn how to put my oxygen mask on before I put on anybody else's." And that's a really hard thing for women to do. We are productive multitaskers and we take care of everyone's, not only physical needs, but also their emotional needs. And the last person you've taken care of is yourself. I think my cancer lesson was learning to say "no" and learning to put myself first. Just the exercise of saying "no" for me was challenging. Sometimes you just have to say, "I can't," and you have to be OK with people being frustrated or disappointed. And I think in some ways it really enhances your real relationships.

Sheryl found solace in journaling—but very deliberately, only writing for herself. She also practiced meditation.

I had a great friend of mine tell me that the gateway to awakening is emotion. And to actually hold an emotion, to experience it, is the only way that you will have lived. If you continue to push everything down and not look at things as they are and at least acknowledge and experience despair, disappointment, joy, love—all those emotions that life deals you—you're just suppressing them. I believe that it surfaces in a health way, or an "unhealth" way.

Part of my experience in life has been to always be busy and to be always working, always getting better. Always growing as an artist, always growing as a writer. And it became, in some ways, a screen. So after I was diagnosed and had completed treatment, I made that commitment to myself to not write and not go to the piano or not go to the guitar or any instrument and make a project out of my experience. Not define my experience by writing a great song or even a poem, but to actually be quiet and to be present and to not go to that thing that I've always used to define myself.

Writing in a journal for me was really hard. I mean, to write, to just be writing and not write to be clever or not write to be great or not write to be giving voice to everybody else in the world except for myself, was really hard. It was hard to sit down with a blank paper and just write. And sometimes I felt like it was just like a colossal waste of time. But I would do it anyway, because those are the moments where you meet yourself.

And meditation has been a lifeline, for a brain that is active as mine is with basically self-imposing judgment—and we all have it. We can be very critical of ourselves and we can tell ourselves terrible things about ourselves that simply aren't true. And meditation, to me, is the tunnel out of that. It's the way to quiet the overactive part of your mind that judges everything. Meditation also helps you to handle what every moment of the day hands you. It elongates the moment and it slows down the reaction. To just give myself those twenty minutes in the morning and twenty minutes at night. Those are my moments of just quieting my mind. And it's a gift I give myself.

■

It was hard to sit down with a blank paper

and just write…

But I would do it anyway, because those are the

moments where you meet yourself.

■

THE COMEBACK

Crow has been cancer-free for fifteen years but still takes her "cancer lesson" to heart.

That idea of controlling what life looks like, that definitely went out the window, as well as this idea that life has a certain way it's supposed to unfold. I grew up in a close-knit family. My parents are still married. I grew up thinking, "I'm a nice person. If I work really hard, good things will happen: You fall in love, you get married, you have kids." And I realized after having breast cancer that the picture that you paint for yourself can be very limiting. This idea of what you think your life is supposed to look like and how it is supposed to unfold can really keep what's meant for you from coming in. And so when I was done with treatment and had a little time away from it, I just decided that life didn't have to be the way that I thought it was going to look.

So shortly after treatment, she began the process of adopting first her son Wyatt, now age thirteen, and Levi, now age ten.

I decided that if I wanted to be a mom, I would start the process. And if it worked out, then that's great. If it didn't work out, at least I rode the boat halfway across. And that's what happened. The next thing I knew, in the oddest of ways, my kids came in.

Nowadays, the hole in her breast left by her lumpectomy gets more and more pronounced. Her skin doesn't bounce back the way it once did. But all of those marks are a sign of a life well-lived.

My body, up until I was diagnosed, was a complete extension of all the things I needed to get done. It was a vehicle. And I just assumed it was all going to work right. And I don't run my body like I used to. I am extremely grateful for the fact that, most everything in my body, as far as I know, is working great. And that's by the grace of God. And that's the same with aging. My car, it's got a few dings in it now. I'm going to embrace the fact that it's still running.

BARBARA DELINSKY

Let breast cancer be the pathway you take toward a better life. And I'm not talking about the hereafter. I'm talking about the here and now.

■ ■ ■

Bestselling novelist Barbara Delinsky, who just published her eighty-fourth book, built a wildly successful career as a novelist by writing, like all writers are told to do, about what she knew. She has written nineteen *New York Times* bestsellers—most of them about the challenges women face every day related to love, marriage, friendship, and personal loss. She developed a devoted fan base through her relatable characters. But for much of her career, one topic remained strictly off-limits: breast cancer.

Even before Barbara was diagnosed herself, breast cancer was a personal demon. Her mother died of it, and Barbara had grown up convinced that she would eventually succumb to the same fate. It loomed so large in her own life that she avoided putting her fictional characters through it, even though, as she later learned, breast cancer would play a big role in strengthening her bond with her readers.

THE DIAGNOSIS
Barbara had her first mammogram when she was twenty-nine years old [in 1973].

My mother had died of breast cancer and I was terrified, quite honestly. It never quite went away from the back of my mind because I remember her final days, and I remember five years of her getting weaker and sicker.

I sought out a doctor who would do annual checkups. This was way before any guidelines were issued. And I really truly expected at some point to have a problem. I had mammograms as often as it was allowed. I had numerous biopsies. I was a basket case before every single mammogram, before every doctor's appointment, because I was convinced that they were going to find something.

I never liked making big celebrations of my birthday. Back then, it was kind of like, "Is this going to be the last one?" I never planned too far ahead. As my kids reached each milestone—Getting done with elementary school. Getting through puberty. Getting into college—I just felt each step was a little bit better for me because I felt like they would be able to take care of themselves when I was gone.

I didn't plan on any great long career because I didn't think I was gonna be around. And I was just having a good time.

It was no surprise to her when, at fifty-one years old, the results of a needle biopsy came back malignant.

THE BATTLE

Barbara had a lumpectomy and went through six weeks of radiation, five days a week.

But unlike Sheryl Crow, who took a break from songwriting during her treatment, Barbara plunged headlong into her writing.

I was fine through [the radiation]. Some people say you get tired towards the end. I don't recall getting tired. I finished one book and started another. When you write the way I write, you live and breathe your characters and your plot. And that's what I did. I simply immersed myself in somebody else's life, not in my life. Was this an escape? Yes, of course. It was an escape of the first order, and I'm very proud of it. It got me through breast cancer in the best possible way.

Then, almost a year to the day later, her doctor found another anomaly on her mammogram—this time in the other breast. She couldn't do another round of radiation, so she decided on a bilateral mastectomy with reconstruction.

The whole thing was a six-hour procedure. I had the surgery and reconstruction in the same procedure. I had to go in to get continually more saline [in her temporary expanders] and then they put the permanent implants in a few months later.

But that was probably the worst experience, medically, in my entire life, because what nobody had told me was that radiated skin does not stretch. It burned. The actual injection itself was painless—they would find the port and pump in more saline—but going home, oh my God, my whole [radiated] side was so painful. I couldn't raise my arms.

We could not do the second part of the reconstruction, in terms of fixing nipples, because the skin was too thin on one side. And I think quite honestly—I can joke about this—the only thing worse than not having nipples is only having one. You think of a wet t-shirt contest. So I acclimated myself to it. What could I do? There was absolutely nothing I could do.

But having had the bilateral mastectomy, and having gotten rid of all the potentially offending tissue, I felt liberated for the first time. I felt like I could look toward a future. It was wonderful.

She was jubilant, but she wasn't broadcasting that jubilance to the world. She hadn't told anyone outside her immediate circle that she had been diagnosed twice, though she did hint at her diagnosis in her sixty-seventh book *Coast Road*.

I did not want people to look at me and say, "Oooh, honey, how are you feeling?" I just wanted them to look at me like nothing was wrong, because in my mind, nothing was. So I didn't say a word. It wasn't until three or four years out from diagnosis and treatment [that] I wrote a book [with] a breast cancer survivor [character]. And her story was very much like mine.

This woman [Catherine Evans] was in her early forties. She was a fun character who had been there, even though her husband couldn't take the whole diagnosis and left. So now she was dating and trying to grapple with the idea of having had a bilateral mastectomy—the sexual ramifications of that whole thing. She was just very upbeat and wonderful and exciting, and readers felt that. And they kept writing to me, so that one book later, two books later, I was still getting reader mail on Catherine Evans.

■

Having had the bilateral mastectomy,

and having gotten rid of all the potentially offending

tissue, I felt liberated for the first time. I felt like

I could look toward a future.

■

THE COMEBACK

So Barbara thought about writing her first work of nonfiction. She started reaching out to her existing fanbase, asking women if they'd battled breast cancer and, if so, what advice they had for other women. Their responses became the basis for *Uplift*.

I thought of doing this book because so many readers seemed to want a role model. And it occurred to me that I could be that role model.

There was no book out there which included the feedback of several hundred people. And I had a platform with my work. This was in 2000. We didn't have social media as you and I know social media. I just sent notes out to my email list, which probably at that point totaled ten or twelve thousand names. I posted notes at Mass General [Hospital]. People came out of the woodwork. What I had asked them for was more positive things. And I got some flak for doing that. I mean, we all know about people who die of breast cancer. Back then, we did not know about many who lived.

I wanted them to tell me their experiences in the most positive light. I didn't want to hear about how awful the treatment was or how bad a doctor was or how unhappy someone is, and I did get those kinds of letters too. I got letters from some people who said, "I'm so offended by this whole proposal because there's nothing good about breast cancer. It is the worst thing that could have ever happened to me." Well, that wasn't what I was writing my book about. I felt so badly for some unhappy people that I wrote back to them. We'd go back and forth, and I was able to get wonderful submissions from them. I'd like to think that they just needed someone to vent to. And after venting, they could think about something that was positive.

I was stunned at the number of people who wrote to me and said, "I've had breast cancer...I was diagnosed ten years ago...I was diagnosed last year." Word spread around. It reached the Lieutenant Governor of Illinois.

The first version of the book had 325 contributors. Its fourth edition, which came out in 2011 to commemorate its tenth anniversary, features 450. Barbara accepted no royalties on the book, using them instead to set up a breast cancer fellowship at Massachusetts General Hospital.

I have spoken at breast cancer events, and inevitably there will be people there who say, "I was in your book." I feel like I know them, and it's been a delight when I bump into people—a lot of whom are happy and healthy and just moving along in life and doing new things. Or even now, I'll get a letter after one of my novels that says, "I was in *Uplift*." I have also gotten a few notes from people who either were married to someone, or had a mother who was in *Uplift* and who subsequently passed away. And that too meant a lot to me because they'll say, "It meant so much for her to be in your book, we feel like it's a lasting legacy."

As for Barbara herself, breast cancer is now more than twenty years in her rear-view mirror. And now, she embraces each birthday.

When I turned seventy, we had a family reunion. It was my three sons, and their wives, and their kids. It was the first birthday I ever remember that I was happy, and upbeat, and totally engrossed.

I think that once you've had breast cancer and you've been diagnosed theoretically with the worst, this thing that could lead to death, well, you're going to do everything that you can do so it doesn't lead to death. But then you have this second chance to be daring. I got a convertible. I never would have dreamed of owning, much less wanting to ride in, a convertible. Because they're dangerous, aren't they? But after breast cancer I got one and loved it to bits. I [also] got a butterfly tattoo. The butterfly is a sign of life. So I think it's about just enjoying life. Let breast cancer be the pathway you take toward a better life. And I'm not talking about the hereafter. I'm talking about the here and now.

KARA DIOGUARDI ON BRCA, IVF, AND BEING PROACTIVE ABOUT YOUR HEALTH

Kara DioGuardi is a Grammy-nominated songwriter, former *American Idol* judge, record executive, and philanthropist. She has written and produced songs for P!nk, Katy Perry, Celine Dion, Kelly Clarkson, Britney Spears, Christina Aguilera, and many more artists. She also runs a boutique publishing company and is a visiting scholar at the Berklee School of Music.

In 2011, Kara was half-watching a story from CBS New York reporter Stacey Sager, in which Sager described her battle with breast and early ovarian cancer, and how she credited genetic testing with saving her life. Kara's mother passed away from ovarian cancer in 1997, and Kara believed that her late mom was steering her toward the BRCA test.

> I saw it and I said, "You know what? That's very similar to my story. I should probably go back to my doctor [in Los Angeles] and tell him I need the test." He didn't understand why I wanted to be tested [but] I insisted that he test me, and they found [BRCA2]. He told me, "I've never had this in all my years. I've never seen BRCA." And I'm like, "Yeah, of course you haven't, idiot. Because you're not testing anyone!"

At the time, Kara and her husband Mike had been trying to start a family. They had already been through eight rounds of IVF.

> Those drugs can't be good for a BRCA carrier, having all those hormones run through you, playing around with estrogen and progesterone. I had had so many IVFs. My fertility doctor said, "You can do one more round, but after that you just need

to get rid of your ovaries." So I did one more round of retrieving eggs and luckily that ended up producing my son [Greyson James], who was carried by surrogate. And then I had [a hysterectomy and oophorectomy]. When I had my mastectomy, he was eight months old.

Many people, including this author, feel that their breasts got an upgrade with their post-mastectomy reconstruction. Kara isn't one of them.

They're the weirdest thing ever. They're hard as rock. They look good but it's just the feel...[But] I kind of looked at it as, "There will be some positives to it. My boobs will be lifted, forever. They're certainly not going to sag. It's going to be interesting when I'm eighty."

The series of events that led Kara to take preventative action to reduce her high risk of breast and ovarian cancer was so improbable and fortuitous that she describes it as a "God wink." Which makes sense. After all, her last name means "watched over by God."

EDIE FALCO

Once somebody says you have cancer, the feeling of
betrayal by your own body is really intense.

■ ■ ■

Edie Falco is a four-time Emmy Award-winning actress who starred in
TV shows *The Sopranos* and *Nurse Jackie*. She is the star of the 2020 po-
lice drama *Tommy* and also starred in the 2017 miniseries *Law & Order
True Crime: The Menendez Murders*.

Edie was diagnosed with breast cancer during *The Sopranos*. Carmela
Soprano may have been a fictional character Edie played, but Edie believes Carmela saved her life.

Acting can be like a dangerous thing because you forget where you end
and the character begins. That happened over the first number of years. I
kept falling in love with my costar and then realizing, "Oh, he's not the
character, what am I doing?!" I was forming sort of inappropriate connections with people when it was really just based on the play. And over the
years you learn the boundaries. But you also know you can get very deep
into actually inhabiting another person, and it's one of my greatest joys in
what I do. It was very helpful to step inside of this other character who
didn't have cancer. She had a husband, she had these kids, she had a lot
of money, and she had nothing to worry about. As my acting teacher used
to say: "Take a little vacation from yourself." And I could very fully inhabit
that for a number of hours a day, and I think it saved me.

THE DIAGNOSIS

Despite her obvious talent, Edie never expected fame—and had a hard
time accepting that she deserved it.

I was a nerdy kid growing up on Long Island, I never fit in. Nobody's
famous in my family history. Trying to become comfortable with what has

happened with me and my career has been a big part of my trip. I loved acting and I knew I'd always do it, but I never knew I'd be able to support myself. I certainly never would have been so grand as to imagine what has happened to me.

You always wait for the other shoe to drop, so [the breast cancer diagnosis] sort of made sense to me. Like, oh, of course. Of course I'll have to die in the middle of shooting this very popular series! I get it. Now it's all making sense.

Edie's experience underscores the fact that doctors, like everyone else, are human beings. Sometimes they don't make exactly the right call, which is why it's so important to go into each appointment as your own strongest advocate.

In the late '90s I felt something. I went in and they said, "Oh, women your age have dense breasts, and it's probably nothing." And the truth is, they were right. It went away [but] since I'm a little OCD, I kept feeling it, because in my mind it was getting bigger.

So here it is, 2002. I felt something. And I was terrified. I went in, and they checked it and said, "Well, women your age have dense breasts. We see it on the mammogram—if you want a biopsy, you can—but we think it's nothing." And that's all I needed to walk away.

So now it's 2003, a year later. And my boyfriend said, "What the hell is that?" And I was like, "Oh yeah. Right." I sort of knew it was still there, but in my mind, it was nothing. It's going to go away just like the other one did. Whatever.

But in September of '03, in the course of a day, I went in for what I thought was a pretty routine mammogram and biopsy. And by noon, I found out I had breast cancer.

On the day of the biopsy, Edie was a nervous wreck, and her doctor was reluctant to give her the bad news.

I first went in to get the mammogram. I was very nervous. It's misery. And I passed out. I've never passed out in my life. [But eventually] they did the biopsy, and it was very painful. Then they said, "You know what? We're not going to have the results yet. You should go to your gynecologist, and she'll be able to give you the results." And I was like, "What?"

It's a very strange situation, to be someone that people know. My cancer doctor told me it's a "celebrity factor." Doctors don't even know they're doing it, but they are more likely to tell you that you're fine. They may even unconsciously skew the results of something because they don't want to be the one to give bad news to you. You don't want to get angry at them. It's a psychological thing. But I think that may have been part of what happened.

So I walked through the city, with my boyfriend, into my gynecologist's office, knowing that something was fucked up. I got in there, and she said they found cancer. And from that point on, you go into a blackout, almost. And thus began my journey.

■

You always wait for the other shoe to drop, so [the

breast cancer diagnosis] sort of made sense to me.

Of course I'll have to die in the middle of

shooting this very popular series!

■

Nevertheless, Edie was able to channel the shock of her diagnosis into some highly emotional scenes on the set of *The Sopranos*.

The morning that I found out that I had cancer, I had to go work on the *Sopranos* set a couple hours later. It was totally surreal. I [called] the producer, who was also my friend, Ilene Landress, before work, and I said, "I was just diagnosed with breast cancer."

Luckily they were scenes that had a fair amount of emotional content to them. They weren't, you know, full-blown anxiety scenes, which is really where I was, but they were high stakes, which was helpful.

This was the season where Tony and Carmela were getting divorced. I remember scenes where I'm carrying groceries outside of a store, and I'm stressed and upset, and I end up dropping the groceries on the ground.

You know, I've never seen the show—I shoot the scenes and then I forget about it. And I remember thinking, it was working well that I was in a place to make this very easy.

I also did a big scene where Jim [Gandolfini] and I met at a restaurant, Tony and Carmela met at a restaurant and had to talk about the divorce. So it was very angry, emotional, cold, and high stakes. And we said some very unkind things to each other.

Edie had asked Landress not to tell anyone else besides *Sopranos* creator David Chase. But Gandolfini, her costar, found out.

I said something about big news, like I just got a lot of big news or something. And he said, "Oh my God, you're pregnant!" I was like, "Oh my God, that's not it!" Talk about a conversation-ender. So I told him, and it was clear that I didn't want it to go any further, and it never did. So nobody knew about it.

THE BATTLE

Edie went to a few doctors, but she ended up going with one who came highly recommended from her friends, who did some research for her. Being a celebrity worked in her favor.

He took me on because he was a fan of *Sopranos*, I have all kinds of mixed feelings about that. I was like, had this been five years earlier, I'd be like everybody else. Sitting in an office, waiting for their next appointment, you know? It's weird.

Ultimately, it didn't matter to Edie whether the doctor was treating Carmela Soprano or Edie Falco. Because her doctor had dealt with celebrities before, he had a plan to keep her treatment discreet.

I didn't care. I knew that he was the best and the smartest in this business. And he said to me, "We have a thing where we hook you up with another patient who's on the other side of it." So he gave me the phone number of another famous person who had been through it.

It was very good to know that there was another person with that variable, somebody who other people knew. I asked about how they let other people know and how did they handle it. It was very meaningful to me.

To have cancer, in and of itself, is a challenge. But to also know that people know details about your life, and apparently care about it for whatever reason—I wasn't born knowing how to handle that stuff. I'm a kid from Long Island. This was a whole new thing.

They were so respectful. They would bring me up back elevators—and the truth is, I never asked for that, because I'm not really that way. In retrospect, I'm glad that they did it that way because I never would have asked for it, but I'm sure it helped me keep it private. At the time, I needed to process stuff on my own, in a small, tight circle with my friends and family.

But celebrity has its disadvantages, too.

[When my treatment was done] *Page Six* called my agent and said, "We heard Edie Falco had cancer, and you gotta give us some details about it because we're going to print it anyway, so you might as well give us the real information." My agent said, "We don't know anything about it." Which is not true, but anyway… So they printed what they knew, which was that.

It was some woman at *Page Six* who outed me. And I was very upset. The fact that it was a woman who did this was particularly insulting. I understand, you want to be the one who breaks the story or whatever, and it's not that much of a friggin' story, but you gotta know that everybody does this their own way. It seemed like such an egregious affront in a way.

I started getting phone calls and emails and people stopping me on the street. And I wasn't quite ready. I mean, I knew at that point I wasn't going to die from this, but it took a little time to process this for me.

I had people stopping me, saying, "Oh my God, I'm so sorry, I'm so glad you're OK." I don't do well with that stuff. It's just weird. It's like, "How do you know about my breasts? I've never seen you before," you know?

Edie first had a lumpectomy. The pathology report came back suggesting that a full regimen of chemotherapy and radiation would be most effective. The whole process took about eight months. Edie worked the entire time. That's not for everybody, but it worked for her.

Once somebody says you have cancer, the feeling of betrayal by your own body is really intense. You find out this thing is growing in your body that could kill you. Even sleeping at night. It was as if you were sleeping with an intruder and they were standing over you.

I said, "Give me the absolute strongest chemo you have. I don't want to go through this ever again, and I'm very strong." So [the doctor] gave me Adriamycin [a drug whose nickname is the "Red Devil"] that actually destroyed the veins in my hand.

Ilene was a master at scheduling my days around chemo so I could go through it and come into work later, or have a day of rest after that. And working kept me so sane. Routine in general keeps me calm. Acting is an insane lifestyle I've chosen, for someone who likes routine. But within that, the more I'm able to stick to what I'm familiar with, the better I feel. So I would go to work, and part of the treatment was steroids, so the steroids would keep me energetic for a couple of days.

It was towards the end of a particularly grueling season, so the cast and crew were doing eighteen-hour days and they looked so much worse than I did. And nobody knew, except we ended up telling the hair guy. I said, "I need the best wig guy around and we gotta get a wig made." We had the wig made just in time for when my hair started falling out. And nobody knew the difference.

I continued to jog, to run. And they would give you the steroid and the next day I would run like, five miles in like forty minutes. It was fantastic. And I made this ridiculous hat for myself. I made a baseball cap and I sewed long hair into it and a ponytail underneath it. And then I'd take the hat off at home and I'd have a bald head.

To see myself with a bald head freaked me out a little bit, so I always wore a little cap at home. I had a million weird little caps.

■

Acting is an insane lifestyle I've chosen, for someone
who likes routine. But within that, the more I'm able
to stick to what I'm familiar with, the better I feel.

■

THE COMEBACK

Ironically, it was her breast cancer that ultimately led her to another
major milestone: the adoption of her children.

When I became diagnosed, my boyfriend and I were talking about kids.
Although we weren't quite there yet, it was recommended that I harvest
eggs. So I did all that, and it was scary because they pump you full of hormones to get a good supply. Meanwhile, my cancer was estrogen-receptor
positive [the cancer cells grow in response to the hormone estrogen] so it
was dangerous to do that. You're hoping that as you're beefing up your
estrogen, you're not giving Miracle-Gro to your fucking tumor.

So then they harvested eighteen eggs. They said I broke a record. I was
like, "Oh, that's nice." I didn't realize you had to fertilize them at the time.
So my boyfriend fertilized them. Long story short, we broke up. And here
I have these eleven fertilized embryos that I couldn't use. So I donated
them to science after all was said and done.

I remember, I was in L.A. and had a specific memory of realizing, "I
think I'm not going to die. I think I'm going to get out of this." And he and
I had broken up at that point, and I thought to myself, the way I've made
any big decision in my life: "Oh, I've got to do this now. There is no right
time."

I'd met Rosie O'Donnell a number of times. She has adopted a number
of kids, and she told me, "If you're ever serious about adopting, give me
a call." That's what I did. She gave me a bunch of phone numbers…A year
later, they handed me a little baby boy—which is unbelievable, that I ever
didn't have these children, that are the biggest thing in my life.

I wasn't with anybody and I thought, "I'm going to do this by myself." I'm not going to like, start dating with the hope that someone will be the father to my kids. I was way more interested in having children than being in a relationship at that point.

When Edie had been cancer-free for six years, her doctor asked her if she'd be interested in genetic testing. She was positive for the BRCA2 genetic mutation, which increases the risk of both breast and ovarian cancer.

[Edie's breast surgeon] said, "We'll just check you every three months." Then I met with a woman doctor. She said, "Don't do that. Get rid of your breasts and your ovaries."

I had already adopted my two kids, I wasn't using [my ovaries] anymore. And she said, "Why would you want to, every three months, go there and panic that they're going to find cancer this time? Get rid of that." And that's what I did, and haven't looked back.

Since the oophorectomy led to an immediate shutdown of estrogen, my memory was really jogged, and I probably won't get it back. My kids tease me about it. They'll say, "It happened like two seconds ago, how could you not remember?" But somehow it doesn't affect my memorization stuff for work.

My genetic counselor said, "Now you have the question of, do you want to tell your family members?" Which I did. And my sister got tested and she doesn't have it. And everybody else in my family said, "We'd rather not know. We'd rather leave it alone." I said, "All right, I've done my due diligence."

When the news first got out that she had dealt with breast cancer, it was hard for Edie to face people who wanted to commiserate. But now, she embraces it. Rather than get spirited up to her doctor through hidden elevators, she walks through the hospital's front doors.

I'm always in for bone density tests, and I go in once a year for my screening and all that stuff. I make a point of going in the front door, hanging out in the lobby. I feel like, to see me there and recognize me, if that's at all helpful to anyone, I would love to feel that I could be of service in that way. I sit in the waiting room. It's like, "Yeah, I'm just one of you guys. And look, you can get to the other side of this."

JILL KARGMAN

I've never been a cleavage girl. It's just not part of my

look. I'm like, granny. I call it "cadaver chic."

■ ■ ■

Jill Kargman is an actress and writer whose work sheds a critical and
humorous eye on a mysterious species with which she is intimately familiar and uniquely qualified to lampoon: the moms of New York City's
Upper East Side. Her 2007 book *Momzillas* was turned into the Bravo
series *Odd Mom Out*. In 2011, she published a memoir in essay form,
written in her wickedly funny style, entitled *Sometimes I Feel Like a Nut*.

Doctors play one of the most important supporting roles in the breast
cancer stories of the women in this book. The majority are compassion-
ate, empathetic, and great at guiding their patients down what can be a
confusing and scary path. But they are also human. And some have more
flagrant—we'll call them *demonstrations of their humanness*—than others. Jill learned that the hard way during her third pregnancy.

THE DIAGNOSIS

Prior to her breast health scare, Jill was no stranger to cancer.

I had a melanoma that had spread to my leg. And you couldn't see it.
Most moles have that ABCDE [asymmetry, border irregularity, color,
etc.]…there are ways to spot it. And mine didn't have any of that. It just
kept bleeding. I was like, "This keeps bleeding." My doctor at the time,
who was a man, said, "You're pregnant, you're being hysterical. Everything bleeds when you're pregnant. Your gums bleed and you're emotional." And I'm like, "Yeah, but I'm kind of freaked. Every time I take a
bath, there's blood on my towel. I don't want to keep doing that. And he's
like, "The second you have the baby, it won't be a problem."

So then I had the baby. The baby was six months. The baby was a year.
Every appointment, he just left the mole. And then, since I knew it was

my last baby, I wanted Botox in my elevens—above my nose, I had these really deep lines. And he's like, "I don't inject poison into people's faces. I'm a medical dermatologist. You need to get what I call a scumbag dermatologist." Isn't that crazy? I'm not sure if he's retired. I mean, he's like 150 years old.

So I went to this mom, a friend of a friend. And she gave me my Botox, and she's like, "Anything else?" And I said, "No, but actually, now that I'm here, I have this mole that keeps bleeding." She's like, "Uh, that's weird. It looks totally benign. I wouldn't worry. But I want to take it off because it's big and if it keeps bleeding, you know, it's in the way. It's in a traffic zone." So she took it off, and then two days later, she called me and said, "I am so sorry but you have a very, very rare melanoma. And you have to go to Sloan Kettering right away. And they're going to have to excise like a whole bunch of this." I had, like, a peanut M&M in there.

I was bedridden. And then I had a cane for six weeks after the wheelchair part. I went for five years for follow-ups and chest X-rays because the cell likes to travel to the lungs. That was no fun either. I had scanxiety all the time.

I have a foot-long scar on my leg. So my kids always see me. You know, I walk around in my undies and they see my huge scar.

Jill was later told she would have been dead in eighteen months if she hadn't done anything. Once it was all over, she and her original doctor—the one who wouldn't do anything about her mole—had a phone conversation.

My parents remained patients of his for like a minute, and they told him and he called me crying. He said, "I'm so sorry." And I said, "Listen, everybody makes mistakes and doctors are human. But I bet you if I was a man, you would've taken it right off." I said, "You used the word hysterical and the Greek root of that word is hysterikos, which means 'uterus.' That's a very sexist word for you to use."

She admits that she had a bit of a God complex when it came to medicine, always putting blind trust in her physicians, never challenging their decisions. But after her brush with death, she resolved that she would still listen to her doctors—but she'd listen to herself first. It wasn't too long before she had to put that maxim to the test.

[Because I had a family history of breast cancer] I started getting mammograms at age thirty-eight per my doctor's advice. I just stayed ahead of it. And part of the reason I did was I went with my aunt to chemo. And I sat with her and I thought, "One day this is going to be me." Before genetic tests were even a thing. My grandmother was dead at forty-six, and I just—this is so weird—I knew my whole life it was coming for me.

From the very first one I got, they said, "Oh this is really dense. You have to do an ultrasound every six months in addition." And I thought, that's fine, lots of people do that. So I just had been doing that for five years. And then one fall, [at age forty-four], they called me and said, "We need you to come back."

[When I went] back they said, "OK so you have two lumps in your left breast. We are gonna have to do a biopsy. We hadn't seen them last year and we want to just check everything out." It turns out they were OK, but they said I needed to do another MRI in three months. So I did the other MRI in three months. And they said, "OK, they're the same size, but we need to do another MRI in three months." In six months, I had three MRIs.

I went back to my doctor and I asked, "Am I doing these MRIs kind of indefinitely?" Because I had an appointment for a fourth in April. And she said, "You know what? I'll be really honest with you. We're gonna have to watch this. And with your family history, yeah. You'll be doing these indefinitely." And I said, "OK, I feel like a time bomb right now." She suggested I get genetic testing. So I sat down with the counselor, and she said, "OK, well, the good news is you don't have BRCA. You have CHEK2 [which functions the same way as the BRCA mutation does, but it is found on a different part of the DNA's double helix]. And so instead of an 80 percent chance that you're going to get breast cancer, there's only a 65 percent chance." I thought, "That still sucks. Those are not great odds."

So I went back to my doctor at Sloan Kettering. She looked at my whole file. And she said, "Look, I'm not allowed to tell you what to do. This has to be patient-driven. But if you were my daughter, between your family history, this gene, and these two lumps, I think your left breast is a time bomb." I was like, "OK, done. Like, I don't even need to think about it." She said, "Take a couple months to think about it. You have until April for your next MRI." And I said, "Nope. I'm not waiting. We're doing this."

THE BATTLE

Jill quickly met with a breast surgeon her doctor recommended.

My husband, he's a really sweet guy, but he's really skeptical, and he sees everything as a business. He said, "Of course this breast surgeon is going to tell you to do it; he's a surgeon." And I said, "He's not going to just like go around chopping people's body parts off to make a buck. This is a very passionate guy. He's a thirty-year veteran in the field and really a renegade. Come with me to the consult."

And Harry ended up being the one who was like, "Oh, you're doing this." And the guy wasn't even trying to convince him. He just said, "Let me just share some statistics about this disease. I have so many patients where, retroactively, we went back [after a mastectomy] and they had CHEK2. There are other breast cancer genes. BRCA1 and 2 are just the most famous. This is a serious gene." My husband, who was [initially] skeptical, asked, "When can we get on the calendar?" There was a fire under his ass.

Together, Jill and Harry calmly told their three children, who at the time were fifteen, twelve, and ten.

We went out to dinner. After we ordered I said, "Guys, I want to just tell you what's going on." I said, "You know how all these people in my family have breast cancer and I've been freaked out. Well, I got this mammogram."

My middle one is very sensitive. Her eyes are huge. They open even wider. And she said, "Was the mammogram bad?" And I'm like, "No, no, no, no, I'm fine. I don't have cancer. But I do have this gene. And I'm at a very elevated risk, and I'd really rather nip this in the bud. So I'm gonna do surgery, and it's gonna suck, and I'm going to be in bed for a week or two, but it's going to be OK. I'm doing it so that I can stick around." And they were like, "Oh, great."

I think a lot of it is how you present it. And [kids] can pick up on fear. I truly wasn't that scared. I had had, weirdly, a number of surgeries for a middle-aged person.

Recovery from her double mastectomy wasn't easy, but it was much more bearable than the debilitating excision on her leg she had just a few years earlier.

I was walking around, like, two days later. Not that I was trying to get an award or anything. And I don't think there's anything wrong with drugs. But I was only on Tylenol because I really have a bad reaction to opioids. The last time I was prescribed them, I didn't lay cable for eight days. I don't know how America's addicted to it. They must be full of poo.

During the surgery, doctors inserted drains in her chest to help clear post-operative fluids and blood, along with small expanders that would need filling every week in order to make room for her permanent breast implants.

The drains freaked the shit out of me. With my leg, I had a really grisly scar, but I got to watch it heal. I wasn't like living with this weird-ass shit, like, fluid pouring out of me.

A nurse showed Harry what to do [to clear the drains]. But he had to go to work in the daytime [so] my mom came over and helped.

This author can attest to the bizarre pain of someone squeezing small plastic globes connected to tubes coiled around your chest muscles. Imagine someone sticking a tiny vacuum through your chest and, as the vacuum turns on, the sucking sensation is accompanied by a barrage of thumb tacks. It's nothing compared to chemotherapy, and it only lasts a few minutes, but it's very strange.

It's really creepy to see fluids from your body pouring out in these bags. My friend sent me this thing called a Marsupial Pouch. It's like a terry cloth belt with Velcro. And then on either side are pockets hanging off. You just stick each pack in there. So you still see the red juices flowing, but it's not the same as seeing these two packs. Looking at those made me nauseous.

Kargman was lucky enough to have more than one friend who took surgical steps to reduce their risk of breast cancer, and who were willing to share their experiences with her. She calls them her "tits fairies."

If you have a good tits fairy, you can get through it.

My first tits fairy is a woman in New York who was a friend's friend. We talked on the phone for an hour. She's the type of person who cuts through the shit, so I knew she would not sugarcoat things.

She sent this huge pillow, that U-shaped thing. And then just all these little texts of encouragement. I sent her my dates, and she put the dates in her phone. I think she was abroad when I was doing my reconstruction in August, and she was like, "Hi, how are you feeling, how's everything?"

My second tits fairy was a mom at one of my kids' schools. I wasn't that close with her but I always liked her when I saw her around. And we actually had to walk safety patrol together in the rain with these hideous fluorescent-orange vests, like, "I'm sure the streets are much safer with us walking around!"

And afterwards, I felt just so comfortable with her. So I broached the subject and said, "Can I take you to breakfast one day after drop-off?" She sent me really funny cheer-up stuff. I couldn't have gotten through it without those two, only because, as much as I leaned on my mom, who came over every day and made me lunch and watched The Thomas Crown Affair, and my inner circle, my five best friends were so there for me, you really need someone to describe stuff to you.

You don't want to be annoying to your doctor, even though they say there's no dumb questions, but I felt more comfortable going to somebody who had been through it. And both those people were prophylactic, so I felt safe, because if it had been somebody like my aunt or my grandmother who were diagnosed with breast cancer, I think I would have felt like I was diminishing their experience by complaining about the prophylactic version.

Kargman's tits fairies also came in handy after a difficult few appointments with the plastic surgeon who performed her reconstruction.

He's really a nice man, he's very well regarded and has done a lot of boob jobs up and down Park Avenue. But I found that he was trying to get me to go bigger than I wanted to be.

And I kept saying "no." If anything, I wanted to go smaller. I was basically like a small D or a big C. And I said, "I wish I could just be like a regular C, if that's a thing, or even a B." And he was explaining I can't do that because then your nipples will point down and whatever. I was like, fine. But then when we were doing the fills, he kept saying, "Well, I want to fill out here, I want to get this dent perfect." And I said, "Hey, I'm not going to be in *Playboy* here. Like, I'm married. I don't care." And he said, "Well, I care. And maybe you might do *Playboy*. Who says you can't?" He was joking around. And then I was like, "No, seriously, this is my last fill." And he's like, "No. Trust me, your husband will thank you for it." And I was like, "Fuck you, buddy. This is my bod."

I was super weirded out by that comment. And it's really not up to him. It's my body. And one of my two tits fairies said to me, "I have a couple friends who have gone to either this guy or a handful of other guys. And they all want to give you full cans, and they think they're doing you a favor, so they're going to give you what they deem to be this aesthetically pleasing, you know, set of melons." But it wasn't what I wanted.

■

If you have a good tits fairy, you can get through it.

■

As an aside, this author wants to underscore that there are plenty of plastic surgeons, and all sorts of medical professionals, who do not act this way. In fact, in this author's experience with implants, her plastic surgeon convinced her not to go as big as she wanted.

I went in for my next appointment and I said, "Listen. I'm going to be really clear right now: You're not touching me. I have a really, really great wardrobe. Not that you would know that because you only see me in scrubs, but I'm not, like, setting my closet on fire, pulling buttons to close a shirt. I wear Edwardian collars. I dress like George Washington. I don't dress like Stormy Daniels." And I had to take a tone, actually. I always respect doctors, but it got heated.

He was like, "I'm just trying to help." And I'm like, "Yeah, I'm just trying to stay exactly the way that I was."

And I thought to myself, what if you're a weaker person? Or strong, but you don't know how to articulate it? I felt like my backbone is steel, particularly after everything I went through. I had no problem pushing back, but sadly, I've heard a couple cases where people are still not used to their boobs, and they feel a little bit bummed that they claim that they told their doctor they wanted a C and they woke up with double D's. And then when they mentioned it to their doctors, they'd say, "Well, we had to for symmetry." And the patients are like, "Why are you trying to be so perfect? Like, Hugh Hefner's not calling me from the grave. What the fuck?" So I think you have to really advocate for yourself. Or if that's not your personality, then bring a friend who can be your loud mouth, because that's a super big bummer.

THE COMEBACK

With her surgeries behind her, Jill is now thinking about what the medical landscape will look like for her children—what options they will have to deal with their potential genetic risk.

One of my doctors said, "By the time your kids are of age, there will be gene therapy." And I don't even know what that is [but] I was like, "Oh, phew. OK, cool." But I think that he thought that I had little kids. I mean, I have a fifteen-year-old who has full breasts. So I don't know exactly the timeline for these alleged medical breakthroughs, but I sure hope that she doesn't have to go through this.

But then again, it still is twenty-nine, thirty years away for her. If you think about twenty-nine years ago, what these poor women suffered with mastectomies…My grandmother just got like two big scars and that's it. They didn't bother with reconstruction. It's a totally different world now. And so for my children I'm hoping it will be as exponential a jump forward.

MAGGIE KUDIRKA

It just helped to know that complete strangers were supporting me and hoping I was healthy and well again. That really helped me get over the fact that my career was over, and that I might have a new career through Bald Ballerina by educating people.

■ ■ ■

Maggie Kudirka is the "Bald Ballerina," who runs a blog and social media account by the same name geared toward sharing her story with stage IV, or metastatic, breast cancer, and providing a resource for other young women dealing with it. She is the creative director behind the annual "No One Survives Alone" ballet concert in Baltimore, Maryland.

At age twenty-three, Maggie had turned the dream of every young American ballerina into her own reality. She had recently graduated college and was living on her own in New York City, training with the prestigious Joffrey Ballet Concert Group, which puts young dancers like her on the fast track to a career on stage.

I was living the life, basically. I had just graduated college and I was living on my own in New York City, doing what every dancer wants to do. And I was living a life like a twenty-three-year-old. I was enjoying it.

THE DIAGNOSIS

Maggie had been in New York City for a few months when, in February 2014, she felt pain in her sternum and discovered a pea-sized lump in her breast.

I didn't really have time to go to the doctor's because we were in re-hearsals all day, and then by the time we got out of rehearsals I was exhausted and didn't want to go to a walk-in clinic or to a doctor. So I just kept pushing it off.

When I first felt the lump, I of course Googled it…and it said breast cancer under age forty is rare. I was healthy, I was active, I didn't smoke or drink, and I wasn't on birth control or anything. So that eased my mind, but still in the back of my mind, I thought, "This could be breast cancer, I should get this checked out, but I don't want to."

Finally, she decided it was time to see a doctor. So she and her mom went about finding one in Baltimore, her hometown. It wasn't easy.

I didn't have a doctor in New York, so my mom was calling all the doctors for me. And they kept saying, "Oh she's twenty-three, it probably won't be cancer. We can fit her in in August." And if I had waited until then, who knows where I would be?

I think my mom probably called four or five doctors before I was able to see a nurse midwife. She was able to prescribe a mammogram, but the doctors kept saying, "No, we'll see her in August."

So by the time I got it checked out [by a physician], you could visibly see my lump. When I felt it, it was probably the size of a pea, and that was in February. By the end of May it was the size of a small grapefruit.

Following her mammogram she had a biopsy, and a week later received the results: She was diagnosed with stage IV breast cancer, which is also known as metastatic because it has spread to other parts of the body. In Maggie's case, the cancer had initially spread to her lymph nodes and bones.

When I was diagnosed, it felt like a dream. I was in this daze for probably a month or so because it just didn't feel real.

I got a second opinion after I was diagnosed. The first doctor, when I was diagnosed, said, "Oh, you can still go back to New York, you can still dance with Joffrey, you will just need to take a day off for treatments." I thought, "Great!" But I didn't have a good feeling going to that doctor, so we got a second opinion, and [the other] doctor said, "Look. If you were my daughter, I would make sure you were home, you weren't dancing 9 to 5. You have to take care of this before you can go back to your career." And that was so upsetting to me because I was on the path to becoming a professional dancer. It was just there, right in front of me, and I couldn't do it anymore.

I burst into tears when the doctor came in and told me. My mom put on a brave face, but I know she was affected by it. My dad doesn't do well with bad news, so he freaked out and [was] diagnosed with gout because of stress. I have two brothers and an older sister. My one brother pushed away, because he's not good with medical stuff…And the other brother stepped up. He was like, "What do you need? I'll help you, I'll take you places." My sister researched stuff for me and made sure I was comfortable during treatments.

◼

I was healthy, I was active, I didn't smoke or drink, and I wasn't on birth control or anything. So that eased my mind, but still in the back of my mind, I thought, "This could be breast cancer…"

◼

THE BATTLE

When Maggie was first diagnosed, she went through six rounds of chemo that consisted of five drugs. Two of them were targeted therapies that she is still taking, and three were actual chemo drugs.

By the sixth treatment, my doctor couldn't feel the lump, and the pain in my sternum that was caused by breast cancer was gone. My body basically took those chemo drugs and ate them up and got rid of the cancer. Before I was diagnosed, I hated taking any kind of pill medicine—I would refuse to take it. I personally think that helped because my body wasn't used to Tylenol or Aspirin or anything in my system. Also, I was still active. I was still dancing while I was doing chemo.

The week after my [double] mastectomy, I was back in the studio. I saw my doctor three months afterwards, and he said, "That wasn't what you were supposed to do." But I felt good enough to do it, and I was careful. I didn't do anything too crazy.

I opted not to get reconstruction. And since I am stage IV, I am required to go for maintenance treatments every three weeks.

My cancer is hormone-driven, so my doctors shut down my hormones, basically, and that's why I'm in menopause. And that's not good on my heart and bones and everything, so it's just like, "Ugh."

Young women with metastatic breast cancer are such a low percentage of cases that we're kind of overlooked. The treatments aren't geared for young adults; they're geared for women over forty, because that's the majority of breast cancer patients. We're not given a lot of options. I'm in menopause, and I'm in my twenties. I'm like, "How is this possible?" And then my oncologist said, "You won't be able to have children. Are you OK with that? Do we need to freeze eggs?" It's just a huge disappointment that the doctors and researchers aren't looking into ways of helping young adults with breast cancer, because we are a growing number. I'm not upset I can't have kids, but many of my friends with breast cancer want to be moms, but we can't adopt because we have cancer, and that's a red flag for adoption agencies.

When she first started this new phase of her life, Maggie had to find ways to fill the hours that weren't consumed by doctors and drugs.

I don't think it was even a week after I was diagnosed, I was emailing my professors from my college [Towson University] and asking, "Hey, can I come take classes?" One of my teachers had taught us to use social media and blogging to promote ourselves, and he suggested, "Why don't you start a blog? I think it would be good for you and a journal of your cancer journey." When I was diagnosed, I thought, "I'm going to be very secretive about it, I'm not going to post it everywhere." But then I thought about how this could be a way for me to keep family and friends updated without getting a million calls and texts and people bombarding me asking how I'm doing.

So I was sitting at the table with my mom, and I said, "I don't want [it] to be called 'Dancing Through Breast Cancer,' 'Dancing With Breast Cancer,' or anything like that." It wasn't who I was. Then I thought, "What if I just called myself the Bald Ballerina?" And it just clicked, and all the domains were free, and I was like, "This is a sign, I need to do it."

At first, her posts were focused on keeping her friends informed about everything that was happening to her. They were all relentlessly positive, just like her.

July 1, 2014: Just finished my 1st round of chemo!!!
Thank you to my mom, and cousin Amber for hanging out with me all day. And to Nurse Terri for making sure I am getting the right medications. Finally to my oncologist Dr. Riseberg for making sure I get the best treatment for my case.

July 30, 2014 [the day she received a wig made with her own hair]: I got my real hair back today! It is my halo. It looks just like my hair because it is my hair!!!!

Then she started receiving messages from other young women going through similar challenges. As Kudirka was developing her own voice, she found herself speaking for other women very quickly.

I get a lot of messages from young women, young moms, about, "I felt this lump," or "My doctor's not letting me get a mammogram, what do you think?" And I always tell them to find a new doctor or really push your doctor to give it to you because you're in charge of your body, not your doctors. And you know your body best, not them, so you need to be the boss of it.

I tell them to live in the moment, not to stress too much about what's in the future, because I don't know what tomorrow has in store for me. I know what I have planned, but I never know what's really in store. And I tell them to start standing up for themselves because it's never too late to do that.

Her blog posts take readers through the ups and the downs.

September 15, 2016: This week, I had my 1st glitch in the 28 months I have been getting treatment. Monday morning I overslept and felt dizzy and weak when I got out of bed. Fortunately, I had scheduled my 1st appointment with my new primary care doc who is wonderful. She found that I had very low blood pressure and a very high heart rate.

I was told to take it easy, drink a lot of fluids, and eat salty things. I am so grateful she didn't send me to the hospital for hydration. Hydration makes for a very long and tedious day.

Dizziness and weakness are side effects of some cancer drugs that I take. It is a pretty scary feeling. What is really scary is that long term use of any cancer drug can affect other organs and cause long term damage. Many metastatic breast cancer patients face the prospect that the drug that stops the cancer can damage the heart, liver, kidneys, etc. I hope that will not happen to me.

In April 2019, she wrote an incredibly vulnerable, personal post in which she showed a picture of herself, bare-chested, her mastectomy scars displayed, and talked about her decision not to have her breasts reconstructed.

April 16, 2019: Recently I have been thinking a lot about beauty and the difference between inner and outer beauty. Outer beauty is something you can easily change and alter. When I first met with my breast surgeon, he asked multiple times if I wanted reconstruction. I stayed firm and said I didn't want reconstruction because my breasts had caused me a lot of pain and gave me cancer. He then asked about romantic relationships. I said I wouldn't want a relationship with anyone who was just interested in my body and couldn't love me for me. I have embraced my scars and love my body now. Inner beauty can't be easily changed. It takes a very long time for someone to change who they are. How you treat and speak to others is a big window to one's inner beauty.

Maggie's first year of treatments cost $334 thousand. Even though insurance covered most of that, her parents still owed more than $25 thousand.

My parents own an auto repair shop—it's a small shop, so it's not like we're that well-off. When I was diagnosed, we knew the cancer treatments would be expensive, so we needed to find a way to raise money and help take off some of that stress of paying the bills and insurance. We started a YouCaring page because we knew about GoFundMe but we did some research, and YouCaring doesn't take any fees. They don't require you to raise a certain amount before you receive the money. They're really supportive of people with medical bills, so we thought it was a good fit. It's just been amazing how complete strangers will donate, and that really just touches me because I don't know these people, and they're really hoping I get better and stay well and not have that stress.

I know I'm past a million [dollars spent on treatments]. I hit over a million in Fall 2018. We joke with the hospital, "Oh, she's giving you guys a million dollars. She should get her own wing." Because if I was a donor and I gave that much, I would have my name on something. Patients don't get that, though.

Maggie gets health insurance through the state of Maryland's public health exchange and receives a federal subsidy because of her low income.

It's always nerve-wracking—I never know if I will get [insurance] because my income is so low. But if I go onto non-private insurance health care, they could deny my drugs. They could deny a scan. They could deny anything they want. So it's really nerve-wracking this time of year to see if I will be approved and will be given health insurance through Blue Cross. Luckily, they've given it to me every year, but it's always just something that we have to worry about. The premiums and out-of-pocket costs and all of that are steadily increasing.

This road has not been an easy one for Maggie to walk—let alone dance—down. In fall 2019, she experienced another health setback.

My cancer returned to the original spots, which were my sternum, spine, and hip. And then it also spread to my femur. At first, I was heartbroken because I had had three years of clear scans. To go in and feel good going into the scan and then come out of it with…not good news, was really devastating for me. I went into a deep depression.

But in the back of my mind, I knew I was still on my first line of treatment. My doctor continued my treatment plan as we were doing and then took another scan three months later to see if it was fast-growing, and what the cause of it was. We read that certain vitamins could possibly feed cancer. So I took a break from some of my vitamins, and that seemed to help. But when I had my scan in September those spots were still active—they were still lit up.

That scan also showed some cancer in her lung nodules. That prompted her doctors to switch up her treatment entirely. In March 2020, Maggie tested positive for a mutation on the PIK3CA gene, which qualified her to begin a brand-new drug designed specifically for people with that mutation. She'll add it to her existing hormone therapy.

Insurance approved it and all of that. I'm just waiting to get it in the mail. I am very relieved that I finally have a treatment plan and can finally start trying to beat this great flare up of cancer.

One thing that helped heal her broken heart: her new Pomeranian, Momma Mia, with whom she now competes in dog shows.

My mom suggested that I get [an] emotional support animal, and Pomeranians are great. They're nice and small. They fit in a bag. Lots of times people don't even realize she's there.

She really has helped me be in better mental state because she always just looks at me so happy and so excited. She loves being a show dog. And it's just a nice thing to do because, when I'm at a dog show, I'm not in the cancer world and I'm not in the dance world. I'm meeting people who have such a variety of backgrounds. I'm not talking about breast cancer and "What are your side effects?" "How are you feeling?" It's so nice to just get away from that.

THE COMEBACK

Since its birth in 2014, Maggie's blog has grown from a way to pass the time to the core of her multifaceted brand, which now includes fashion shows, film, and work with breast cancer awareness campaigns.

It's kind of cool that my story is still relevant because, I mean, I'm five years out of my diagnosis. So for me to still have such amazing opportunities come my way, even though I'm not bald and I don't "look sick," is really exciting for me. I've gotten to go to L.A. I went to the Tribeca Film Fest. It's just crazy how many opportunities I've gotten, because for me, it's just my life. But to others, I'm an inspiration.

She's also been producing—and starring in—an annual fundraising concert called "No One Survives Alone."

For a time, I worked at a dance studio, and one of the moms had breast cancer. She was like, "I think we should put on a fundraising concert for you. It will just be something fun for the girls to do." So I started planning it, and it just gives me something to do and keeps me busy. It raises a lot of money for my medical bills. And so many dancers from New York come and dance, and every year we get more and more professional dancers.

Today, Maggie is as positive as ever, focusing on gratitude. And it rubs off on the people who visit her blog and social media pages.

January 1, 2020 [comment from Barbara D.]: Wishing you health, nothing else...hugs from Slovenia and keep dancing!

November 6, 2019 [comment from Georgia W.]: Stay strong, you are a mighty warrior and one of the faces of this disease that says I refuse to give up. Thank you.

October 31, 2019 [comment from Colleen P]: You are beautiful inside and out. You are such an inspiration to all of us. ♥ ♥ ♥

JACLYN SMITH

When they said "cancer," I wasn't going to let a minute
go by. And boy, did I go to town.

■ ■ ■

Jaclyn Smith is a Golden Globe-nominated actress and businesswoman
who starred in the original *Charlie's Angels* TV show. Her eponymous
lifestyle brand has grown to include fashion, home decor, cosmetics, and
wigs.

THE DIAGNOSIS

Jaclyn was busy maintaining her lifestyle brand and helping her daughter get ready for a summer dance course in New York City when she
received her breast cancer diagnosis in 2002.

I went in for a yearly mammogram, and the radiologist said, "We might
feel a little something. We don't think it's anything, so don't worry, but we
want to do further tests." So I went back in, and I did a core biopsy [in
which an entire core piece of tissue is removed from the breast, as opposed to a fine needle aspiration which removes only a few cells]. The way
they were doing it was more stressful than the surgery itself. I was up-
side-down on a table, and they were taking little slices of my breast and
photographing them, and running from one room to another. When I came
back a few days later, the first thing the nurse asked me was, "Did you
come alone?" And I said yes, never even thinking, because I was so
healthy, I felt so vibrant.

The doctor came in and said, "I have some good news and bad news…
You have breast cancer, but it's very small and we've caught it very early."
And I know the first thing I said: "Am I going to be here for my children?"
And he said, "Absolutely, you're going to be here for your children."

But I started to panic, and I said, "I want to meet the surgeon today,
I want a mastectomy." He said, "Well wait. Let's not jump the gun." And

I said, "No, I already know, I trust your judgment, just bring in whoever you think is good, I'll meet him today, and I need to move on."

At the time, my daughter had gotten into a summer intensive dance program in New York, and I didn't want her to miss it. I didn't know what I was talking about.

So I got back into the car and I called my husband [Dr. Brad Allen], who was practicing in Chicago. He commuted on weekends. And I said, "I have breast cancer." He said, "You must be mistaken." I said, "Brad, I have breast cancer. And I'm gonna get a mastectomy, and we're planning it now."

He said, "First of all, wait. I need to talk to the doctor." And I said, "Nope, I've made the decision, I'm doing it." And he said, "Well I'm going to call the doctor now."

After he consulted with the doctor, my husband said, "Look. The studies show lumpectomy with radiation in your situation is as effective as a mastectomy." He talked me into the right choice, because I talked to other people who also said [the same]. It was not a big tumor.

Jaclyn was at peace with her decision and was eager to move forward. She wasn't stressed out about the treatment. She was, however, worried about telling her children.

When they say it's a disease for the family, it is a disease for the family. The whole family reacts in a different way. My son, who believes everything I say, and if I had said I could catch bin Laden at the time he'd probably believe me, said, "You'll take care of this and you'll get it out, and everything will be OK, Mom, right?" And I said, "Yeah, absolutely." My daughter, on the other hand, not a good story: She struggled. She refused to go to Alvin Ailey and do the summer intensive.

Jaclyn's husband tried to be stoic, but his behavior betrayed him.

I love movies. [Brad] doesn't always want to go but...once I was diagnosed, he would say, "Oh, let's go to a movie." "Can we see another one tonight?" I said, "Brad, what? Two movies in a night? What's going on?" I think he was overcompensating for it a little bit. I always say my husband lives on the other side of Disneyland because he's so positive—and he is, and he's a non-alarmist—but he did have a hard time.

THE BATTLE

Jaclyn had a great support system between her family and friends.

[Brad and I] lived apart at that time, so I had my friends, and I had my mom and my brother. Brad flew in the day of the surgery, but he's a pediatric heart surgeon and was working out of Chicago. And I never once went to radiation by myself. Not one time. When I speak on breast cancer, I talk about the power of girlfriends and how they saw me through and how they would pick up the call, and drive me here, drive me there. That was a very positive part of me going through the treatment. I didn't do it alone.

Jaclyn would sometimes get a little tired after her radiation sessions, and they did make her skin a little red, but none of it stopped her from being active. In fact, she picked up her pace.

I did a cameo in the *Charlie's Angels* movie. I did a semi-regular role on [CBS crime drama] *The District*, and I launched a furniture line. It was almost like, when they said cancer, I wasn't going to let a minute go by. And boy, did I go to town. I was going to turn down *The District*. I thought, "I've done a series for five years, I don't know. Do I really want to go back and do series television?" And oh my God, it was so good. Craig T. Nelson is one of the most talented actors I've worked with.

I worked through radiation and *District* let me off if the time was conflicting with a scene I was shooting. I'll never forget that. That's the kind of support you want, for them to say, "OK. We'll work around it. We'll shoot another scene, and come back after your treatment."

As much as [cancer] was frightening, it gave me a new lease on things. And as I've always said to my children, go towards the fear. Go out on a limb—that's where the fruit is. So I went towards the fear.

She hadn't planned on "going public"—telling people outside her immediate family and closest friends—but then someone leaked the story to the media.

> They sold the story and made money on it. It was so disturbing. And it makes you question, who did this? You think, "Was it the hospital? Was it the doctor's office?" This was unfair, to take someone's sadness and make money on it. The story itself was positive. They wrote, "She handled this with uncommon grace" or something like that. But I wasn't ready to tell the world. And I needed to get stronger in order to talk about it. And it certainly wasn't good for my children.
>
> And I just wasn't ready to talk about breast cancer. I wanted to learn all my facts, I wanted to get through my treatment, I wanted to still be normal. And then I have people call me and say, "I just can't believe you have breast cancer." Well, what does that mean? Like I'm going to die in a minute? It's not an easy subject when people don't know how to talk to you.
>
> And I think some of the most effective things were a quiet note from somebody. "Sending you lots of love and all positive thoughts. Love, so and so." "You'll get through this, I'm here if you need me." Something like that.

■

As much as [cancer] was frightening,

it gave me a new lease on things.

■

THE COMEBACK

However difficult going public was, however, it made her realize how helpful her story could be for other people.

> It made me realize that you need to talk about it, and it helps you to support somebody else. I think I'm a compassionate person, but now I

give lots of time to a stranger. They come up to me and [say], "Well, my mom, she was diagnosed." I'm a highly emotional person, so all of a sudden, they're my best friend. I'll say, "OK, let's talk about it." We'll talk about whether the chemo put sores in their mouth, and things like that. I'll tell them my husband's a doctor with research. That kind of thing. I think it makes you enjoy life in a different way.

Jaclyn found other ways to help, beyond talking to strangers who approached her. In 2013, she partnered with celebrity hairstylist José Eber to create a line of wigs. Every year, they visit cancer patients and give them makeovers.

In October, we go to City of Hope [Cancer Center]. José takes his team, we go out there, and we do a day of beauty on women, young and old, who are going through chemo, who have lost their hair. I can't tell you how powerful that day is.

José knows women—he knows what looks good. The wig line donates the wigs, and they're cut and styled to the shape of the women's face, and we take pictures, and it's really a beautiful day. I went into wigs as a fashion statement, but really, when you think about it, when you lose your hair, it's devastating for a woman. It just takes your femininity; you don't feel beautiful. These wigs are really very affordable, so I'm really happy that I can contribute in that way.

With her cancer almost twenty years in hindsight, Smith is still as vigilant as ever, going for not just annual mammograms but alternating them with MRIs, to be sure that if there is a recurrence, she catches it early. Another part of her routine has always been prayer.

It has always been important to me, and my grandfather was a minister, but I think after cancer, it's almost like I wanted to be on my knees for prayer. It just made it more, like, "Oh my God, I'm here, and life is the best!" All I can say is life is so precious. I never finish the day without saying, "Thank you God, thank you for getting me through this, thank you for making me braver than I was, thank you for sparing me other things that I could have had to go through."

SARAH SUSANKA

No matter what people think, you are on your own journey. And don't let anybody tell you what it's going to be
like.

■ ■ ■

Sarah Susanka is an architect, author, and the originator of the "Not So
Big" theory of residential architecture, which champions "better, not
bigger" homes.

Decades before the Tiny House movement went mainstream, before
HGTV introduced viewers to the open-concept floor plan, and before
Instagram turned the Danish word "hygge" into a #lifestyle, Sarah was
exploring the psychology behind these now-ubiquitous phenomena.
This was just at the turn of the millennium, when more was more. It was
the age of the "starter castle." The McMansion. She was asking why people usually congregate in the kitchen, rather than the formal dining
room, and why people are typically drawn to cozier spaces, not grand
and spacious ones.

The answers Sarah found to these questions became the basis of her
bestselling, ahead-of-its-time series, inviting the housing world to focus
less on square footage and more on spaces where people really want to
live. Quality over quantity. That didn't mean a small or tiny house—just
one that didn't have to be so big.

It might seem self-evident now, but it was a revolutionary idea at the
time. And when she published her book in 1998, it made Sarah an over-
night sensation.

I was actually sort of at the peak. *The Not So Big House* [her first of her
series] had come out in 1998, and I had been projected into an entirely
new world. I had been on *Oprah*, I had been on *Charlie Rose*. Everybody
who was thinking about residential architecture was reading my books.
And it was really heady stuff.

THE DIAGNOSIS

Then in 2001, a not-so-big lump near her armpit shrunk her world into a grain of sand.

I found it through a regular self-breast exam. And the reason I recognized it was because, when I was in my late teens, my gynecologist gave me a little bag with a little lump in it, and she said, "This is what breast cancer feels like." So I had that little bag for years. I don't know where it went. But when I felt this thing under my arm, I thought, "Oh. I know what that feels like."

The doctor I originally went to said to me, "We can do [just] a biopsy, or we can take out the tumor at the same time. Which would you like?" And I said "Yeah, get it out of me. I don't want it in there." Then she got back to me the following day, and told me, "Well, the biopsy did reveal just a little bit of cancer." And I thought, "Oh well, that's probably not a bad thing." And so I announced this to my husband to our front porch while he was working in the garden, and it was like I had hit him with a brick. His face turned completely white. I hadn't fully received the news. But he received the news. I mean, he was experiencing for me what I hadn't really let in. And it took me a little while to really grasp the severity of what was going on.

Sarah's cancer turned out to be stage II, which denotes a lump greater than 2 centimeters in size and/or that the cancer has spread to at least one lymph node.

I just didn't really get it, honestly, until I went back to the surgeon's office and went for our first appointment. I had lived a life that was super busy. "Not so big life," no…It was very big. I was a busy author and public speaker, and I had my plate incredibly full. So I'm sitting in this waiting room, and I thought, "These guys, they're just not on top of things. I've been sitting here for 45 minutes!" I finally went up to the front desk and said, "Look! I've got a place to be in 25 minutes." And a woman behind the desk said, "Let me have you talk to a nurse practitioner for a minute." The nurse practitioner came to me and said, as nicely as she could,

"Honey, your life is about to be turned upside down. This is going to be normal. Drop everything you don't have to do off of your schedule and prepare for *you* to be your priority for the next..." I don't remember how many months. She was telling me, "You're not getting the picture. This is not the way things happen, and you can't live as if it is."

And she said, "There are a lot of people who are really struggling for their lives. So there's going to be some waiting, and you're going to get used to waiting. It won't be efficient, and that's the way it is."

It was the first place where I really understood what it means to let go. Some of the language I use in *The Not So Big Life* is to "be obedient to the situation." Here, I had to be obedient to that situation. I was not in control. I didn't have a choice.

In my professional life, I'd been successful from pretty early on. From twenty-one on I was really busy. And I was really good at what I did and was proud of it. So [the cancer was], I think, a contributor to the wakeup call which told me, "You can't live like this. It's not possible for a human being to live at this speed and this intensity." When I became famous through the *Not So Big House* series, I said yes to everything because that book had gotten me to where I was in the world. But you can't say yes to an avalanche. You're going to get buried. I didn't know that, and this is what made me aware of it.

THE BATTLE

Part of learning how to be obedient to the situation meant focusing on accomplishing whatever immediate task or challenge was in front of her, like a round of chemotherapy, and to not try to mask the feelings that accompanied them.

It's the experiencing of this moment: Today, sadness is being experienced. Today, no energy is being experienced. This moment, frustration is happening. Whatever it is, this is what you're experiencing. It's like what that nurse told me in the waiting room: "This is your life right now, this is how it is, so live it and live it completely." Experience what it's like to be in the waiting room of life. And it's not "fighting." It's actually being receptive to what's happening. It's a real different attitude. For me, it was really a question: What will this teach me?

I noticed after my lump had been taken out that all of a sudden, I started feeling angry. I didn't know why. And suddenly it occurred to me: Could that lump have been like a sort of capacitor with some stored emotion, but when it's not there, I didn't have that ability to avoid it? It was so antithetical within my family of origin to even admit that there was anger. You couldn't even broach the subject.

So I looked up, what is the correlation between anger and cancer? And here's what I found: "Extremely low scores have been noted in numerous studies of patient with cancer. Such low scores suggest suppression, repression or restraint of anger. There is evidence to show that suppressed anger can be a precursor to the development of cancer and also a factor in its progression after diagnosis."[1]

In that moment I decided, "I'm going to learn, how is it that I'm suppressing my anger?" And that became a huge part of my healing. When you've got something really repressed, it's almost impossible to recognize. A big part of my own process has been to notice where I hide things from myself.

I had to be obedient to that situation.

I was not in control.

That self-awareness also helped her make definitive choices about her care.

The first oncologist that I went to was a man. As he was speaking, he was telling me the statistics about my chances for survival. And what I realized was that he was telling me that there was a strong possibility I wouldn't make it.

Beliefs are like germs. So when somebody that you have put in a position of authority is passing along a belief of theirs, you internalize it, and it becomes your truth, too. He doesn't mean to—he was just telling me numbers. But what I was hearing was, "You have a good chance of dying from this."

And that sent me into a tailspin of terror. I was so scared when I came out of that meeting, it took my husband, who's a counselor, three days to dig me out. He had to actually reconstruct my belief in life. That's how dangerous it is. And doctors do not usually understand it. I knew this man had my best interest in mind, but he was not the right guy for me. What I knew in that moment was, "I cannot work with this man, not because he's not a good physician, but because his belief is so strong that I'm in danger of dying, and if I get into a rapport with him, I can't keep myself healthy and keep my own integrity going through this process."

So then I started to look for the kind of oncologist that would be supportive and not focused on statistics. And I found somebody, and I am so glad that I took that extra time to do the research to find the right person.

In architecture, I always tell people, "You've gotta have not only a talented architect but somebody that you can really feel connected to, who really gets you." It was the same thing. And she was terrific. And I felt all along like I was being supported through the process rather than constantly reminded that, geez, you've got a life-threatening disease and you might die.

That experience just made me aware of how critical it is that our humanity be there. And I've told so many people since then, "No matter what the numbers say, you are not a statistic." It's enormously important. If you take away somebody's belief in life, they may not even be very sick, but they'll die because they've fallen into a hole that they don't know how to get out of.

Directing the selection of her medical team was one new way in which Sarah could exercise some amount of control over her life when she had lost so much of it. But she couldn't control her response to her treatment.

I was given a choice for chemotherapy: I could do a regimen for three months that would be more intense ["dose dense"] or I could do one for six months that would be not as intense. I decided to go for the three months intense, because I wanted to just get it done. And it was really hard. It's the hardest thing I've ever been through. I was so sick. I'm the kind of person who, when a package says "Take two pills," I take one because I'm sensitive to medication. And it just knocked me flat. I had no energy. I hear about people working through breast cancer treatment. I have no idea how they do that, but they don't have the reaction that I did because I was just flat.

The hardest things are little things that you don't even think about, and most people don't even know about. For example, right after the chemo, the day after, is really tough. You're throwing up; you just feel horrible. And then it gradually abates until the next one. The hard part is that you know, going into it, what you're going to feel like tomorrow.

My white blood cell count went way down, so they give you a shot that helps boost the white blood cell count, but it hurts your bones. Your bones ache. And I can't even tell you, I've never had anything that painful. And sometimes I even had to give the shot myself on the weekends. So I know that I'm putting something into my body that's going to make me hurt so badly. It's so difficult to describe to people you are voluntarily stepping up to the plate to be hurt.

Pooping is incredibly painful because not only does the chemo kill all the cancer cells, but it kills anything that regenerates, which is your whole digestive tract. It's tough! And it's hard to talk about.

But Sarah discovered solutions to help her through it—both mental and physical ones.

I wasn't worried about surviving, interestingly. Once I got past that first oncologist, I didn't think anything bad was going to happen. I just thought, "I have to get through this."

I was forty-four when I had [estrogen-receptor positive] breast cancer, so I got slammed into menopause because they turn your estrogen production off. So I didn't have pre-menopause; I went from full-on to full-off. So I can't honestly tell you how much I experienced was chemo and how much was menopause. But it was intense because I could not sleep to save my life. I had horrible insomnia. And nobody could help me. I'd tell the doctors, and they'd just sort of smile at me, but they didn't know what to do. And it's terrifying when you only sleep a couple of hours a night, and very superficially at that. But I discovered that antihistamines put me to sleep. I discovered, "Oh! All I need is a Benadryl, and I go to sleep!" My life changed that day. It doesn't work for everybody, but it worked for me.

■

No matter what the numbers say,

you are not a statistic.

■

The emotional changes were challenging to reckon with.

I often said during that period, "I don't recognize myself." I didn't feel like myself. My thoughts weren't like my own. I was angry a lot, I felt upset a lot, I felt misunderstood, I felt hurt—all kinds of stuff I had never felt, ever!

One time I did a public speaking event after I had had chemo but I was still really dragging. I got to the airport and they wouldn't let me through to the gate because I was one minute past the cutoff time to board. I fell on the floor in tears. Buckets of tears. I had no coping left. And I suddenly realized, this is how it feels to just not have any resources. You can't dig deeper. There isn't anything more. That was a really powerful lesson, and it allows you to understand people's plight in a very different way.

THE COMEBACK

In a roundabout way, chemo, and the dreaded "chemo brain," actually ended up helping Sarah with her writing.

I remember the first public speech I gave, at least six to eight months after I finished chemo. I remember going to the talk knowing that I used to be able to just talk, like I am right now. Ideas come, I talk about 'em. But my brain didn't work like that anymore. I could only say what I had already said in the past and knew how to say. It was not apparent to anybody in that audience, I don't think. But I knew there was not one ounce of creative thought in it. It was all regurgitated from things I remembered. And I had a very profound awareness in that moment, like, "Wow, I didn't realize how much I depend on that access to whatever's coming to mind in this moment to make that talk work."

That feeling lasted about a year and a half. And it was profoundly shifting. In the middle of all of this, too, I wrote a book. I wrote *Home By Design*, which was, interestingly, very successful. My editor tells me, "The reason, Sarah, that it's one of your best books is that you couldn't write a lot. So you had to be very succinct." I would write a sentence, and I couldn't tell if the sentence made sense. Literally, I was that "chemo-brained." So I would have to do my best. My husband encouraged me just to write a little bit every day. If you only write two sentences, that's OK. Just do it. It's a very important lesson in life: Things happen, even if they're happening at a crawl, you do get there if you step forward.

PART II

THE
EXECUTIVES

THE WOMEN IN this chapter held top leadership positions at their companies, but they were all diagnosed at different times in their business careers. Some, like energy utility CEO Mary Powell, had already reached the pinnacle of leadership when they had to confront their breast health. Others, like haircare guru Chris-Tia Donaldson, were still in the process of building their start-up companies.

Regardless of how mature their businesses were when they were diagnosed, they all had to figure out how to keep their companies afloat while also looking after themselves. And no two women had the exact same strategy. Many took leaves of absence, which made it easier to focus on their health but which forced them—many for the first time in their careers—to hand over the reins.

But even if they weren't physically in the boardroom during their battles, their health challenges had the side effect of helping them connect more with their employees. Battling cancer also gave many of them a new perspective on why they did the work they did, and why they loved it. For others, cancer was a reality check that life is too short, and maybe it is time to take those vacation days and spend more time with family and fewer late nights at the office. In the case of Daily Greens CEO Shauna Martin, a frightening diagnosis led her to a successful second career that she continues to juggle with metastatic breast cancer.

Breast cancer is a difficult challenge regardless of your professional environment. But the women whose stories are contained within this chapter believe that their battle has only transformed them into better business leaders.

CHRIS-TIA DONALDSON

Once you decide, "I'm going to work out. I'm going to go for a walk. I'm going to check this email." Those are little victories. Those little mental victories become huge in terms of your body's ability to fight this disease.

■ ■ ■

Chris-Tia Donaldson is the founder and CEO of the multi-million-dollar natural hair and skin care line Thank God It's Natural. She is also the author of *Thank God I'm Natural: The Ultimate Guide to Caring for Natural Hair*. Her business originated, as so many successful ones do, as a solution to a problem she herself encountered when she was just starting out in her first career as a corporate lawyer.

I started work in corporate America in 2003. The world was a very different place then, from a technology standpoint and an ethnic diversity standpoint. When I graduated from law school, there was this pervasive belief that has been long-held amongst black women that curly hair was unprofessional. When I started my first law firm job, I didn't want to straighten my hair anymore. I wanted my hair to be curly, but there were no products on the market to support that. And in the process of figuring that out, I had to wear a wig in order to look professional, because I thought, "OK, I want to be successful here, I want to look like Clair Huxtable from *The Cosby Show*." And it backfired. I wasn't able to be my authentic self at work...So I started my own company.

THE DIAGNOSIS
By the time of her 2015 breast cancer diagnosis, Chris-Tia had built TGIN from a DIY operation in her kitchen to a full-blown business, with deals at big-box retailers like Target.

I had found a lump in my breast while showering, and I thought for a few months that it was going away or getting smaller, that it must be hormonally related. I did not necessarily feel it was a cause for alarm, but after four months of it still being there, I went in at the urging of a friend. My doctor's office scheduled my appointment for three weeks out or a month out, but my friend really pressed for me to go, and as a result I went to the gynecologist right away. She did a physical exam, and she said, "No big deal, this doesn't feel like cancer, but let's just order a mammogram to be safe." And it turned out it was.

I was shocked. Because I was thirty-six, I'm black, and the example of breast cancer that you see promoted throughout the media, particularly when it comes to celebrities, are Sheryl Crow, Melissa Etheridge, Julia Louis-Dreyfus, Christina Applegate. None of them look anything like me. I felt very alone and very scared.

But from a professional standpoint, it was the best year of my life and the worst year of my life. My career reached almost kind of a pinnacle, even though it's still on that upward trajectory right now.

I never gave up on the company. This is going to sound crazy, but people call this company my baby. It's literally like my child, in the same way a woman who's diagnosed with breast cancer has three kids and she still has to put food on the table. It was like, "I have a company to run," and it wasn't an option for me not to run it. Just because you have breast cancer doesn't mean you stop being a mom or a CEO. So that's how I looked at it.

Chris-Tia couldn't help but notice how, in medical situations, a person's socioeconomic background and race can really affect their psychology in the exam room—and potentially their care.

When I went in for my initial screening, it was at a community hospital on the South Side of Chicago. And anyone's who familiar with Chicago knows it's highly segregated, and it has a higher concentration of lower-income communities on the South and West Side. I went to this community hospital because that's where my OB-GYN referred me to and where she delivers babies from.

When I came back for a follow-up, I was like, "OK, no big deal," assuming this is nothing. But when I got the diagnosis, I looked back on the kind of clients they served, and it was poor Latino and black people, and I thought, "I've got to get out of here if I want to have a chance of saving my life." Without any question, I had to get to Northwestern, which is one of the top regional hospitals but is located on the Gold Coast [an affluent residential area]. And a lot of people don't have that option, whether due to lack of resources or lack of education, and lack of transportation can also be a part of that.

Those differences in resources aren't only evident on the patient side, though. They can also affect how doctors approach patients, as Chris-Tia noticed when she went for her follow-up at the community hospital.

It's not like I wear the fact that I went to Harvard twice on my sleeve, or that I'm a lawyer or that I run a company. Sometimes people's inherent biases come into play. When I came back for my follow-up biopsy, I had all of these questions, like, "What size is the tumor that you're seeing? Is it irregular? Is there architectural distortion? If you had to rate it on a BIRAD scale, what number would you give it?" And I could tell the doctor was taken aback by the level of research that I had done, the depth of my understanding, while still limited, and how aggressive and proactive I was.

Some patients view the medical profession and say, "Whatever my doctor said, I'm gonna do." And I didn't have that attitude. I could tell that she was used to dealing with people who were a little bit more submissive and less aggressive in terms of challenging the process, or questioning what was going on.

Following her own experience with breast cancer, she established the TGIN Foundation to advocate for women patients experiencing financial difficulties.

THE BATTLE
Chris-Tia is a confident woman who is not afraid to speak up for herself. And as she found multiple times throughout her trial, her strong sense of self made all the difference in her treatment.

I'm a lawyer by background; I work in a career field where you're just aggressive. And whether it's something or nothing, you say to yourself, "My friend thinks this is a cause for concern, so let me take care of it." And I bring that up because sometimes patients from lower-income backgrounds or lesser education, get told, "You have to wait a month." And they wait a month. They're not going to go back and push because sometimes they don't have that same sense of entitlement.

In the course of being treated at Northwestern, Chris-Tia never forgot the faces of people she saw in the waiting room on the South Side.

I thought about, over nine months of being treated, little things like paying for parking every day. Paying for an Uber every day. Not having to worry about childcare. Not having to worry about taking time off of work. People think that "cancer = cancer treatment," but there's a lot of social and economic factors that contribute to people not being able to be on their regimen. They may think, "I can't take off of work today and go to chemo," or "no one's going to babysit my kids," or "I can't afford my medication." I didn't have to make those choices.

While she never sat her small staff at TGIN down to explain to them what was happening, they were still a powerful source of support for her.

I think some of them were able to figure it out based on my social media. But they were extremely supportive and having a great team in place was critical for us keeping this thing going. Even though I was going to all these meetings, I still was working at 30 percent. In that year our revenues doubled and the number of stores we got into increased fivefold. We went from around a thousand stores to five thousand stores that year.

Following her surgery in March 2016, Chris-Tia prepared for eight rounds of chemotherapy. But she always thought of herself as a CEO first who was battling cancer, not a cancer patient who ran a company.

When I found out I had to have chemotherapy and I was going to have to go through all of this, I was like, "OK. There's only one meeting that matters." It was a meeting with Target on March 22, 2017, an update meeting. So my doctor scheduled my initial chemotherapy visit so that I would look good for it.

In the meeting with Target I was so scared, even though I'm normally super confident and I present really well. But I go in, give my presentation, and they're like, "Now THAT'S how you give a presentation! That's the best presentation we've seen all day." And then after this Target meeting, we started getting calls from Whole Foods, Sally Beauty, Walgreens, Rite Aid. It was the craziest thing.

That moment fueled me because I had to tell myself—and I tell other cancer patients this—I had to stop viewing myself as a cancer patient. I had to view myself as a daughter, a sister, a friend, a CEO with cancer, and not let cancer be the defining characteristic for myself. I'm this person who enjoys listening to R&B music, watching TV shows, reading good books, making products. And by the way, I have cancer. I let it be a footnote versus my headline.

I had chemo every other week, so I'd be down a week and then up a week. And when I was down a week, I'd say, "I'm kind of checking email, but not really." And then during the weeks when I was up, I just really tried to enjoy being "up," whatever that meant. It might mean going out with friends, but from the perspective of running the company, it meant I had to make the most of being up.

I didn't go into the office for two months. I might have gone over there when people weren't working, if I needed to get stuff or whatever. But the first four treatments I had, the Adriamycin [the notorious "Red Devil"] was the worst. But once I went back in to the office, once I turned the corner on that second round of treatment, I was like, "OK. I can do this." Because that set of side effects wasn't as crazy as the first set.

■

I had to stop viewing myself as a cancer patient. I had to view myself as a daughter, a sister, a friend, a CEO with cancer, and not let cancer be the defining characteristic for myself.

■

THE COMEBACK

For Chris-Tia and her team, her cancer was just another hurdle to figure out how to surmount.

My attitude towards my team was, "This is just another challenge." For example, one time I was in Africa and our manufacturer went into bankruptcy, and all our stuff was going to be lost for a period just as the company was taking off. I've had people quit on me the day before we launched in Walmart. My attitude has always been, "Figure it out."

And when I was back in the office every day, it was never like, "Oh, we need to talk," or have a team meeting about my breast cancer. It was just kind of like, "OK. Back to work." Not even back to work, though. It's funny. One of the girls who works for me said, "You know, you told us, 'Now I'm back.' But you never left."

THE PINK FUND

When Molly MacDonald was diagnosed with breast cancer in 2005, it was the second time in her adult life that her world had been turned upside down in an instant.

The first time was in 1997. She had been living an idyllic life outside Detroit with a smart, rich husband, and five beautiful children.

I would say we were the "3 percenters." I gave up my career in 1985 to raise children full-time, and in the fall of 1997, I drove up the driveway to our beautiful home and saw a note on the front door, about the size of a wrapped card, and read that our house was going to be auctioned off in thirty days.

Her husband had gotten involved in some shady financial dealings, and had put his family $15 million in debt. He had forged Molly's signature on their tax returns, so they were coming after her too.

She arranged a deal with the IRS such that she would not be liable aside from having all their cars repossessed. She soon filed for divorce from her husband, receiving no money in the settlement.

Luckily, she had a plan. Over the years, she'd experienced a sort of premonition that there might come a day when all the money was gone, and she was ready. She liquidated her life insurance and an IRA she had begun when she was single and working at the *Detroit Free Press*. She had all her worldly goods appraised and sold, transitioned her children from private to public school, and looked for work.

Life had knocked her down, but she had gotten right back up. She started working any job she could: selling Mary Kay cosmetics, writing catalogs for school auctions, and doing freelance work for the *Detroit News*. She married a wonderful, supportive man and eventually found full-time work in graphics sales.

By 2005, Molly felt like she had climbed out of the hole her ex-husband had pushed her in. She had just successfully pitched a company on letting her open a Detroit-based branch of their business.

Then, following a routine mammogram that picked up something unusual, Molly had a biopsy done. While she was in New York City, trying to generate business for her new bosses, her doctor called her with the results: she had early-stage breast cancer.

I felt I had to tell these new employers that I had this problem and I didn't feel it was ethical for them to make an investment in me at that time. So, we agreed not to move forward, and now I don't have a job, I don't have any savings, I have no child support, no alimony, a co-premium of $1,300 a month, and an awesome self-employed husband whose business had been tanking.

I was in foreclosure and bargaining with Ford Credit not to come get my car. Every fifty-eight days I pulled that cancer card out and I told them, if they took my car and then I lost my house, then I didn't know what was going to happen.

I met with a social worker, and I didn't qualify for any Medicaid. I didn't qualify for cash assistance or food assistance because it was predicated on my previous year's income, which disqualified me. Friends are delivering food, so we had some food, but by the end of the [cancer] treatment we had no food because when you stop treatment, they stop delivering. So I ended up at a food bank, which was probably the lowest point I've ever felt as someone who had a fine education, an upper-class upbringing. I once had what the world considers everything you need. Now I'm in line in the basement of this church at the food bank to feed my family.

Everything was beginning to unravel. And to be honest, I felt like I wished I had end-stage disease cancer because then I could die and get out of this mess. I had purchased a half million-term life insurance policy so that my kids would have something, at least, if I died. I'm pretty practical.

I met a lot of other working women in treatment who were experiencing similar financial troubles, what they call now "financial toxicity." They were plowing through what retirement funds they had, through their savings, they had very long-term treatment protocols: Whereas mine was six months, some of theirs were a year to eighteen months. They knew that their treatment was going to outlast their Family and Medical Leave Act (FMLA) leave, so they're probably going to lose their job. Now they're going to have a gap in unemployment—how do they explain that? It was just a complete perfect storm of cancer-and-career. It was a shitstorm.

In most health care systems, you can make payment plans for treatment, and if you want to negotiate your health payment, it could take months. But if you can't pay your rent, you're going to face an eviction very quickly. In sixty days, your car is going to be repossessed. Once you start losing these very basic necessities of life, we know that patients make decisions based around that.

The data bears that out. A 2017 Pink Fund survey of 562 respondents found that 41 percent of patients had altered or skipped their medication or treatment due to financial constraints.[2] Another survey found that 60 percent of patients had missed or arrived late to a doctor's appointment because of trans-portation issues.[3]

> *I thought, "Somebody has to do something about this."*
> *Women are adjusting their treatment; they're not taking their*
> *medications they're prescribed, they're skipping diagnostic*
> *tests; some of them are stopping treatment to go back to work.*
> *So I took $50 and bought a book called* How to Form a Nonprofit
> Corporation. *I couldn't get help so I was going to give help.*

The night before one of Molly's two surgeries related to her di-agnosis, she and her husband cast her bust and covered it in gold paint. An artist friend drew battle ribbons across the chest. They turned the bust into her new nonprofit's unofficial mascot and be-gan doing "Bust Stop" speaking engagements in her area.

> *Every Rotary club, women's group, Optimist's Club, men's*
> *group, schools, church basements, synagogues—anybody who*
> *wanted a free speaker—I went in and told my riches-to-rags*
> *story and what I was doing. We officially launched October 2,*
> *2006, with a story in the* Detroit Free Press. *My husband and I*
> *were so excited we couldn't sleep that night because we knew*
> *it was going to be on the front page of the paper.*
> *Little by little, donations started to come into the bank where*
> *we opened an account. And then we assembled a board of di-*
> *rectors which, of course, was anybody who would warm a seat.*
> *At the same time, the reality of my circumstances kind of fell*
> *away. I did rescue the home from foreclosure by going to my*
> *mother and asking for money, and I was able to keep my vehi-*
> *cle, although my credit report tanked.*

Over time, and with a few big-time partnerships including Ford Motor Company in 2012, Molly took her group national. Known as The Pink Fund, her nonprofit organization provides financial sup-port to breast cancer patients to help them meet basic needs, de-crease stress levels, and focus on healing.

Today, we've paid out more than $3 million in bills to patients' creditors. We work out of donated office space; we have a paid staff of three. There are other tiny organizations who will send gift cards or gas cards, or they'll give people money, but we don't do that. We pay their creditors, because the real domino that causes everything else to fall is job loss or an unpaid leave of absence.

I brought my thinking from, "Poor me, who's going to help me?" to "OK, I'm going to fix this." Not fix so much as make a difference. Other people would look at me and say, "You're in line at the food bank. You don't have a full-time job. Your house is in foreclosure. How can you help anyone else?" But the key was I believed I could do it.

SHAUNA MARTIN

When you meet a young survivor, it's almost like you're immediately bonded like you're sisters. It's that immediate of a bond.

■ ■ ■

Shauna Martin built a successful corporate legal career before getting diagnosed with breast cancer. Following her treatment, she turned her hobby of creating healthy green juices into a business, and is now the CEO of Daily Greens, a nationwide brand.

But when she was diagnosed with breast cancer at age thirty-three, Shauna didn't know that the disease was eventually going to lead her directly to her life's passion and a thriving second career.

She was just focused on surviving.

THE DIAGNOSIS

Shauna was working at a small law firm in Austin, Texas, and was breast-feeding her son, who was almost a year old, when she got the news.

At the time I could almost tell through the breast-feeding process that I had a lump that just wasn't going away. I went in to see my OB-GYN, and he said, "Oh yeah, I feel a lump but you're thirty-three years old. It's gotta be a clogged milk duct. But if you're worried about it, and you have time to check it out, here's a prescription for an ultrasound." So I just threw it on the seat of my car and let it sit there for about three months. But it definitely wasn't going away. So finally, I went in, got an ultrasound, and you should have seen the look on the face of the ultrasound doctor. I knew, "Oooh, something's wrong."

And before I could even get out the door of the radiology clinic, my doctor called me and said, "I'm so, so sorry that I did not take this more seriously." He said, "You have to go right now for a biopsy. Like, right now."

I went for my biopsy on my son's first birthday. I had to leave the biopsy office and then throw him a birthday party.

Shauna was diagnosed with stage IIB breast cancer. It had extended to her lymph nodes and was growing aggressively, but had not yet spread elsewhere in her body.

My OB-GYN later told me, "Because of you, I changed my practice completely." This was fifteen years ago. The incidence of breast cancer in women my age was so minimal. It is really on the rise now, and it's quite an issue, but it was really rare. I just think it was a very, very good learning experience for him, and he has caught some really serious breast cancer in the years since, because of me. If you look at the statistics, the rates are going down overall but not in young women. It's actually really scary how quickly it's growing in young women under the age of forty.[4]

Following her diagnosis, Shauna called her sister and urged her to get a mammogram right away.

■

When I called her, I said, "The doctors are telling me you should get checked out. We're sisters, I'm young, this is highly unusual." And she said, "You know, I have been feeling this lump." Three weeks later she was diagnosed with breast cancer too.

■

When we were growing up, we moved around a lot and encountered some really nasty stuff. We are military, so we lived in some weird places. We lived in Puerto Rico for four years, near a banana plantation that they would spray down with pesticides every day. We lived in El Centro near the border, where they used to do some nuclear testing in the desert.

We're not high-risk for anything related to cancer. So the general conclusion by most of the doctors was that we just got exposed to some pretty massive pesticides or other environmental poisons when we were little girls.[5]

■

My OB-GYN later told me, "Because of you,

I changed my practice completely."

■

THE BATTLE

Before she began her treatment, Shauna wanted to do everything she could to maximize her chances of having another child.

I was making plans to have another baby, so I was very unhappy at the fact that the doctors said, "Nope, no more babies for you." So the first thing I did was fertility treatment to preserve some embryos, and that took about two months.

My breast cancer was estrogen/progesterone positive; fertility treatment jacks up your levels of estrogen/progesterone. It's not a healthy thing when you have active breast cancer. There's a breast cancer protocol where they inject you with letrozole (a drug that treats breast cancer in postmenopausal women) and keep your hormone levels steady...but fifteen years ago, this did not exist in Texas. The only guy back then who administered it was a doctor in New York. So I got him on the phone with the premier fertility guy here in Austin, Texas. So I was administered my fertility treatments in Austin but supervised by the doctor in New York. And I was able to harvest eggs and create twelve embryos.

What we should have done is hired a surrogate right away, but we didn't. We wanted to see if maybe I could do it naturally, but I was never given an opportunity to do so. The cards were never in my favor. When I was forty, right around the time when I would have been allowed to go off my tamoxifen, they thought I had ovarian cancer and they had to remove my ovaries.

I waited for two months before I started my chemotherapy. I had three attempts at a lumpectomy, but they never could get clean margins, so they stopped. I did a year of chemotherapy and then I came back at the end of that and did a double mastectomy.

Shauna was the breadwinner in the family, serving mainly one client at her law firm. She worked through her entire chemotherapy treatment.

I would do my chemotherapy on Friday, I was usually kind of down for the count through the following Monday or Tuesday, but about Wednesday, I was ready to get back up and start working.

Chemo was like the worst tequila hangover you've ever had, but for five days. For me in particular, they never could seem to manage my toxic symptoms. I lost thirty pounds. I survived by eating avocados. They were the only thing I could keep down. I had severe nausea. They stopped the chemo a couple times because my white blood cell count would get too low. I thought the chemotherapy was going to kill me.

There were lots of days where I would just work from home. I had a really good set of girlfriends, and I had a one-year-old at this point. So usually one of my girlfriends would come to town and take care of me so my husband Kirk could take care of my son. Then in the second year, when I had all my breast surgeries, I couldn't be left at the house alone with my son when he was in his crib because I couldn't pick him up out of his crib. I finally bought this stepstool, and I would say, "OK. Time to get out!" You know how most kids are climbing out of the crib? He wouldn't. He was a rule-follower. He wouldn't climb out of the crib.

Because Shauna couldn't do some of the things new parents are expected to do, her son grew to look to his father, her husband, for the sort of emotional support that is oftentimes considered, for better or worse, a mother's domain.

To that point, Mom had done all the breastfeeding and kind of done all the heavy lifting, but when I got sick, my husband had no choice. I could barely make it into the bathroom and sit there and supervise the bath time.

That always really bothered my mom. I remember one time, we had gone back home to Arkansas for my grandfather's funeral. I was right in the middle of chemotherapy, and my son needed something, and so he went running to his dad. And my mom was so upset about it. I said, "You know, Mom, it would be so much worse if he only would go to me. Please take comfort that he views his father as an equal parent, capable of taking care of him at the age of one." My father's a pediatrician, so he kind of jumped into the conversation. He said, "Oh, yeah, men are just as good as caretakers of infants and children as women are." It's not a gender thing.

I'll never forget that conversation. I took such comfort that my son's father was an equal caregiver and he was happy to get the same kind of nurturing from his father as from me, because there were a couple years where I was just so unable to be a full mom. I mean, it's sad. I feel like I missed out on a lot because I was in such a fog for a couple of years. But it definitely made my husband a better dad.

At work, Shauna tried to keep her cancer diagnosis low-key.

I was a partner in a law firm, so I basically went to my partners and said, "I'm going to keep my biggest clients and keep them happy, but I need you guys to take over the rest of my clients." And they were happy to do so.

I really didn't tell a lot of people, particularly at work. I just kept it pretty quiet until I started chemotherapy and I was bald. Then I had to start explaining. I had a big legal job and it was very, very upsetting to men, in particular, to sit there with me bald. They would just break down and cry. They just couldn't handle it. I don't know exactly why, but breast cancer hits a lot of men really hard.

So I would wear a wig just to make everybody comfortable around me.

Following her chemotherapy, Shauna faced a new challenge, which is common for breast cancer patients after their treatment ends.

When you're doing chemo, you go to that really strong place inside yourself and just sort of warrior it out for a couple years. I would say the hardest time is when it's all over, and you're like, "I've been in battle for two years. Now what? How do I deal with life now?"

It takes a very long time and a lot of counseling, from my perspective, to get over your fear of dying. You're pretty convinced that you're not going to live. And it takes a very, very long time to shake the feeling that you might die tomorrow, or the next year.

In addition to counseling, Shauna empowered herself by learning how to take advantage of the healing powers of food.

After two years of super-toxic treatment and so many surgeries, the doctors would always look at my sister and me and go, "Oh my God, I would just pray that both of you make it for the next five years. The odds are not with you here." Even on paper, we did everything we could—we definitely increased our odds from 50-50 to 80-20, from the chemotherapy to the surgeries and everything we've done—but he said, "Statistically, both of you probably won't make it for the next ten years." That didn't sit well with me. I had a young child. I also wanted my sister to stay alive too. So I started researching the connection between food and disease. And I thought, "Wow. There's something here." I became convinced that we should, number one, never eat anything that wasn't organic as far as produce was concerned, and that we should be more plant-based. And then I read Kris Carr's *Crazy, Sexy Cancer Tips*. She had one green juice recipe in there, and I thought, "I'm gonna try it!" And it was amazing. I thought, "Wow. I felt really different when I drink a green juice."

So I started cleansing, but I couldn't stick with a straight-up juice cleanse. I was already so underweight; it just didn't work for me. But I could stick to a cleanse when I added food to it. I would add raw, vegan food, which digests very quickly, so you can get right back into fasting mode. I made up my own cleanse, and I would do it once a month for four or five days. It really worked.

And then in between cleansing, I would just be plant-based. Sometimes I would eat raw or raw vegan, which is really hardcore when you're traveling. But through time, I just felt better and better and rebounded, and then at some point I realized I had way more energy than I had had in my twenties. And by the way, when you eat the way I eat, you don't have to work out like a maniac to stay skinny. I would work out maybe twice a week, very moderately. But I could also pick up my bike and ride 100 miles if I wanted to. It just keeps you very lean.

I'd make 32 ounces of green juice a day, and everybody called it my "pond water." Everybody made fun of me. This was before juice bars would even make green juice.

◾

I took such comfort that my son's father was an

equal caregiver and he was happy to get the same

kind of nurturing from his father as from me, because

there were a couple years where I was just so

unable to be a full mom.

◾

Shortly after she started juicing and doing cleanses, Shauna switched jobs. This was pre-Affordable Care Act, which made it illegal for insurance companies to raise rates on people with pre-existing conditions.

I could be the poster child for Obamacare. There was a point where I was completely uninsurable. By me staying on my small firm's plan, I made the cost of insurance for the entire firm unattainable. I had to get off my firm's plan so that the rest of the firm could maintain affordable insurance. For a while, Kirk's company provided insurance, since it was small, but within just a year it was also unaffordable for us, with premiums of $3–5K per month. I had no choice but to leave my firm.

I went to work for a big corporation, so that we could have health insurance. For six years, I commuted from Austin to Dallas, four hours away.

Finally, once insurance companies were no longer able to discriminate against people like Shauna, she was able to return to work at her small firm in Austin. It was during this time that she started thinking about making a career change.

I took the summer off and thought a lot about, "If there was one thing I was really passionate about and that could change the world, what is that?" And I felt so burdened about how unhealthy our country is. It just makes me so sad, every day. I knew that I wasn't going to get everybody to be vegan, but the one habit of mine that I felt like I could share with everybody and actually does make people healthier was drinking a green juice every day. So I started researching the technology around mass producing green juice and making cold calls to figure out where the closest HPP [high pressure processing] machine was to me. At midnight one night in 2012, I made sixty bottles of green juice and took it to the farmers' market the next day, and it sold out in minutes.

And the next weekend I went to another farmers' market, and then within about a month we were in some local retailers, and then within about four months we were in Whole Foods, and then within our first year of business we were nationwide with Whole Foods. We now have national distribution with Costco, Target, Sprouts, and a lot of other retailers.

Shauna's story is one of perseverance and creativity in the face of hardship. The tools she gained during her first bout with breast cancer helped her be resilient when, in 2017, it returned.

They say you should replace your implants every ten years, and mine were twelve years old. So in a routine surgery, I had gone back to replace them. It's standard protocol to send all tissue of a survivor to pathology. About two weeks after the surgery, my doctors called me and said, "Oh, my God, there's cancer in there again." So I quickly went back to my oncology practice, and we started the process of full diagnosis. It took me probably six weeks to get fully diagnosed.

There's a PET scan, a brain scan, a bone scan, a bone biopsy. And then they can decide what the plan is. After doing the fourth scan, the bone biopsy, it was understood that mine had metastasized to my bones. It was the same cancer. It started from a single cell almost all the way up at my collarbone, so out of the radiation range, out of the double mastectomy range. One single cell had reignited and filled my entire chest cavity again. And then it had metastasized to my spine, my hips, and my femurs.

So first they went in to surgically remove as much as possible. Having just replaced my implants, they pulled everything out again. It actually took two surgeries to remove all the cancer.

Shauna actually had a very dramatic time getting into the operating room for the second surgery.

My plastic surgeon went in with us to a breast surgeon, and the breast surgeon did not get it all. It was still all in my skin, my chest cavity, my muscles, everywhere. And the breast surgeon was willing to give up. And then I developed an infection two weeks later.

I had a 104-degree fever. My son and I Ubered to the hospital, and my plastic surgeon met me there and took me in for emergency surgery. He literally made a crayon drawing based on the pathology report, and he kept me there in surgery until he got it all.

He and I both look at the infection as a gift from God. If I hadn't gotten an infection, he wouldn't have probably had the opportunity to bring me in for emergency surgery. He would have had to overrule a breast surgeon to get back in the operating room, because he's not the breast cancer expert; he's a plastic surgeon. And after the first surgery, both of the doctors noted, "Oh, her white blood cell count is so low right now. And her red blood cell counts are so low. Surgery, not a great thing. Maybe we just move on to radiation and hope that gets it." The surgery was risky. What if I'd started bleeding out? My red blood cell count was plummeting. But given the massive amount of infection, my plastic surgeon had no choice. He had to go in. He cared so much. He had gone in, found my pathology report, memorized it.

Following that second surgery, Shauna began treatment.

Then I proceeded to a full chest wall radiation and spine radiation and went on to the least invasive protocol chemotherapy. It's actually not even called chemotherapy; it's aromatase inhibitors, estrogen or hormone blockers. Combined with bone marrow blockers, it inhibits your bone marrow growth, which keeps the cancer from growing in your bones. I can't run anymore. But I do get to work out maybe once a week if I have the energy.

I'm finally reconstructed after two years. My final surgery was in May 2019. But I will be on chemotherapy for the rest of my life. You have to keep changing the medicine up. Usually it gets too toxic after a period of time, and they have to lower the dose. Then it finally stops working. It will be an ongoing thing. I'm very blessed over the course of the last two or three years, life expectancy for my situation has changed from five years to fifteen years, as a result of this new targeted therapy that I'm on, so I still work full-time.

The main medication is oral. But there are monthly supplemental infusions of other medicines and stuff. So I usually go in once a month, see my oncologist, get my meds, my shots, and infusions. It's a whole day, usually. And then I'm able to do scans quarterly.

Sometimes I get my blood worked up more frequently, like every other week, just to check for deficiencies. But overall, they consider me an outlier because I'm very high functioning for the medicine that I'm on. I still carry on with life as if nothing happened. Most women in my situation don't work.

THE COMEBACK

Shauna's work at Daily Greens continues to fulfill her professionally, but the juices themselves have also helped her remain active.

I feel so blessed to be part of a thriving brand. And in order to continue on with a normal schedule, I've just made lifestyle choices. I don't drink alcohol anymore, and I've ramped up my Daily Greens quota to two or three bottles a day. I am very vigilant about my plant-based diet. And sleep is very important. I track my sleep, and I make sure that I'm getting one and a half hours of REM sleep and deep sleep. I used to be the queen of working out [but now] it's very focused and effective, and I'm not wearing my body out by overworking it.

Her biggest priority is her son, who is now fifteen.

I've got three and a half more years with him in high school. I want to make the most of that and be really present for him. I will probably never see him have kids. I'll be lucky to see him graduate from college. It's very difficult.

He does really well with it. I'm just trying to make sure he has a normal childhood.

We don't talk in terms of life expectancy, because I don't know. Just since the time I've been diagnosed, my life expectancy tripled. But he has to take care of me sometimes. Sometimes I come home from work and all I can do is fall asleep on the couch, and he's gotta help me make some dinner and then help get me to bed. I try to shield him from doctors' appointments and chemo and that kind of thing.

She also recently went through another major life change. After fifteen years of marriage, Shauna and Kirk divorced in 2017.

I was married to a wonderful man, a wonderful father, for fifteen years. I think the cancer was this major theme of our marriage and pretty traumatic to the overall marriage.

Sometimes, the cancer was a blessing. It brought us together. But sometimes it was just too much. I needed to go change the world. I needed to make lemonade out of lemons. For my husband, I think he would have preferred life to settle back to normalcy. And it just was never normal again. He was also involved in helping me start Daily Greens, and I think that kind of thing also takes a very big toll on a marriage. Now, we live three blocks apart from each other. We have 50/50 custody of our son. He goes back and forth between us. I consider us to be pretty well-adjusted co-parents.

It was just time to call it, you know?

She believes that her first bout with cancer at such a young age enabled her to maintain a positive outlook.

The statistics were not good. There was a very high likelihood that it was going to come back in one of us [sisters], so I had a lot of time to think about it. I always kind of thought it would be me. My cancer was more advanced than hers when it was first diagnosed. So I had a lot of time to get used to the idea that this was a real possibility for me. And I'd lived my life for the last twelve years as if it would happen.

I always have looked at [my early diagnosis] as a blessing. I mean, at a very young age, I was forced to face my mortality. And people are not often given that gift at such at a young age. And I've made the most of life. If it ends tomorrow, I've had an amazing life. I've lived three lifetimes, I really have. I have no regrets.

I'm entering the phase where I've done pretty much everything I want to do. Now, I think, "How can I maybe leave a legacy and continue the story for others?" And my story seems to inspire people, which is wonderful. How can I transform that into something that's tangible for them? For me, it always comes back to food. It's magical to see. And so it's still my platform. I think it always will be. It's been fourteen years now since I discovered food as medicine. And I'm as passionate about it today as I was fourteen years ago.

Daily Greens is now a wildly successful company and over the years has donated a portion of sales to the Young Survival Coalition, a group dedicated to young women fighting breast cancer.

The drinks each have seven servings of greens in them. Leafy greens are blended with lighter greens and tasty accents like watermelon and jalapeno, with names like "Elevate," "Renew," and "Vitality." Customers can pick up the same juice that Shauna originally started making simply to nurse herself back to health. It's now her "Purity" blend.

ZOLA MASHARIKI

I called everybody and I'm like, "It's not cancer, yay!"
So they asked, "What is it?" And I said, "I don't really
know."

■ ■ ■

Zola Mashariki is a consulting producer for One Community, an independent social impact and film production company. She is the former Executive Vice President and Head of Original Programming for Black Entertainment Television (BET). Prior to that she was the Senior Vice President at Fox Searchlight Pictures, working on such films as *The Best Exotic Marigold Hotel* and *The Last King of Scotland*.

As a successful TV and movie executive, Zola had access to the best doctors and cutting-edge care when she was diagnosed with breast cancer in 2015. But that didn't mean she had an easy journey. Luckily, her community—her own flesh and blood, as well as the family she made for herself—rallied around her in a way that has shaped her life ever since.

THE DIAGNOSIS
It began when her newly hired personal assistant realized after seven months that she had never seen Zola go to a doctor's appointment.

I was working twelve- to fifteen-hour days. And she said, "This is crazy. I'm going to schedule all these doctor's appointments for you. You're just going to do it, and I'm going to make sure nobody interferes with that time."

I think a lot of us women kill ourselves doing ten times what we need to do at work, and then for women of color, we are told by our parents, "You've got to be ten times better, work ten times harder, ten times longer." We service everybody else and put ourselves last.

During her well woman visit, the doctor performed a clinical breast exam.

> He said, "I'm sure it's nothing, but I definitely want you to get the mammogram. There might be a lump there, there might not be, but we just want to make sure everything's OK." Now I know that in cancer speak, it's code for "something might be wrong."

The day of the mammogram arrived, and the perpetually overscheduled Zola was running late. However, she believes her tardiness played a key role in her catching her breast cancer as early as she did. Usually, this doctor sits with the patient to interpret the images, but because Zola arrived late, her doctor didn't have time to do a full visit.

> The doctor was actually with another patient, so she said, "Go get your mammogram, and as soon as you're done, your results won't be back yet but I'm going to ultrasound you, so at least I'll have a sense [of Zola's breasts]."
>
> They don't normally ultrasound you. And the ultrasound is actually what showed that I had some abnormal cells there. My mammogram came back clear.

Zola later learned from her mother that dense breasts—whose irregularities often show up only on ultrasounds, not mammograms—ran in the women of the family.

> This doctor did the same thing that the other doctor did. She goes, "I'm sure everything is great. I'm sure everything is gonna be awesome." And then she leans out of the room and shouts, "Cancel all of my appointments!" And this was after they had told me she had to leave. So I'm like, "What is going on?" And she says, "I know this is totally fine, I see this all the time and there's nothing wrong. But we should do a biopsy right now. I'm going to give you some anesthesia…"
>
> And I'm thinking, "What?! I'm supposed to go back to work!" I couldn't believe it. My doctor was lovely, she talked through it all [while] getting out these massive needles and preparing me for a biopsy.

But the confusion did not end after the surprise biopsy.

My doctor called and said, "The good news is, it's not cancer." And I said, "Oh, well that's great." And she said, "You have something called LCIS [lobular carcinoma in situ]. We have to go in and take out the whole tumor and see if it's the tip of the iceberg, because maybe there's something else. But go ahead and take Christmas break off, and then when you come back I'll remove the tumor. I'm sure everything's OK."

It all happened so fast that I wrote it down. So I called everybody and I'm like, "It's not cancer, yay!" So they asked, "What is it?" And I said, "I don't really know."

Medically, the doctor was correct. LCIS is the growth of abnormal cells in the milk glands of the breast. But it is a marker that suggests a patient is at an increased risk in either breast, in any location, for the development of an invasive breast cancer.

Zola's biopsy took place close to Christmas, so the doctor told her to take some time and go for her pre-planned trip to Florida and Spain. Zola might have physically been on vacation, but her mind wasn't.

Florida was my first stop, and that's where I did all this Google searching. All the information was the same: You gotta take it out because it could be invasive cancer.

I don't know how other women experience it, but I just felt like Alice in Wonderland. I was thinking, "I don't know what happens now. Am I gonna die?"

Also, I redid my will—that was an experience. I'm a single mom, and my twins were four years old. When you think about the person that you want to raise your kids in the abstract, it's different than what's of value to you when you really think, "Oh my God, I actually could die now." When I first did my will, I chose somebody who could provide for them and who shared my values and could give them the upbringing that I wanted them to have. But when I was first diagnosed, I realized that I wanted them to have *parents.* That having a guardian when you suffer your first heartbreak, and crying in a guardian's lap is very different than crying in your mom's lap. And I wanted them to have a mom or a dad.

So immediately, before I continued on to Spain, I spoke to dear friends who I knew had also been trying to have another baby. They had a kid already that was my kids' age, and they shared my values. I asked them, if I died, could my kids call them Mom and Dad?

The one thing I could do [on vacation] is figure out who were the best doctors in L.A. for this sort of thing. My assistant helped me, and at the very least, when I got back to L.A., I knew that I was going to meet with the top breast surgeons, because, as grateful as I was to the first doctor for finding the cancer, I wasn't loving the "it's not cancer" thing.

I went with Dr. Kristi Funk [of the Pink Lotus Breast Center], who was so transparent and amazing and smart, and she gave me every ounce of information that I ever needed, so I could make really smart decisions all the way through.

THE BATTLE

Following Zola's lumpectomy, the pathology revealed a second, more invasive cancer in her other breast. She was given a short window to receive radiation treatment, but it was determined that a double mastectomy would be just as effective.

Before the surgery, she had to find a cosmetic surgeon to perform her reconstruction surgery. She started with a well-regarded L.A. physician, but the accolades that had brought her into his office quickly disappeared in Zola's mind when he opened his mouth.

He showed me pictures of people he'd worked with and was like, "Yeah, this black gal, I gotta show you what I do to black gals." It was…I don't even know what to say.

And then when we talked about money, he said, "I need you to know: I don't know if you're an insurance person, but I'm not the insurance guy." He was implying that if you mention insurance to him, you are not his clientele. And insinuating that I am an "insurance person"…I think so much of it was loaded and gross and awful and terrible.

But the final straw was when he tried to make Zola promise she'd be OK if he couldn't preserve her nipples.

He said, "You might end up with nipples, but I'm not going to commit to that." What I thought he was wanting to do was have me sign off on a lesser standard of care right away. I kept going to other doctors, asking, "How come this doctor says he can't save my nipples?" They would say, "We don't know what he's talking about."

Mashariki quickly found an excellent plastic surgeon who didn't ask for a pre-surgery ultimatum and would perform a nipple-sparing mastectomy, which allows a patient to preserve her nipples. That procedure requires what's called a nipple delay, in which a surgeon disconnects the blood vessels from the nipple in order to force it to find new sources of blood flow. But Zola quickly experienced complications.

Two days after the nipple delay [an outpatient procedure], I took my kids to school, and as I was dropping them off, I noticed that my breast had grown to the size of a watermelon—not a small one; a big one! So as I'm walking my kids to class, I'm watching my breasts grow and grow and grow. And I'm freaking out, but I know I can't freak out in front of them. So I shove them into class, and I get back to my car and start driving home.

As I'm driving, I call the doctor and she says, "Don't even go into your house. Come straight to the facility." So I drive myself there, I walk in the door of her office, and I just collapse. From then on, I don't remember anything that happened because they took me straight into surgery. I had passed out.

The cause of Zola's complication is still undetermined. At the time, she wasn't just worried about what was happening to her body. She was worried about her children.

As I'm driving to the doctor, I'm calling my kids' godfather to tell him I think I'm going to be out of commission because I didn't know what was going to happen. I said, "If she takes me in surgery, I don't want my kids to be at school and they can't contact anybody." It was one of the scariest days I've had.

Zola ended up having eight procedures in total: her biopsy, her two lumpectomies, a surgery to prepare her for the mastectomy, the double mastectomy itself, her implant surgery, the nipple delay, and the corrective nipple procedure. That was a lot, over the course of a year and a half, to recover from. So following several of her surgeries, she went to an aftercare facility once she was discharged from the hospital. These are popular in Los Angeles, especially for plastic surgery patients looking to for a discreet place to recover, but aftercare facilities and home care options are available all over the country. For Zola, it was a safe place to spend a few days before going home.

My doctor had recommended it for recovery, but another part was really for my kids. I had had so many surgeries that year that when I came home, my kids really wanted to be close to me. So if I was in the bed asleep and I was taking painkillers, I would often find a kid curled up under me. And they wouldn't know that they were causing me pain.

Many of the doctors were male, and they kept saying things like, "You'll recover in two weeks." And I guess, maybe that's the physical healing time. But the amount of time that it really takes your body to heal, it's not just two weeks. There's the question of how long it takes for a scar to heal or stitches to dissolve. And then there's another aspect, which is, what does it take for you to have the energy to get through a day?

So aftercare was amazing for that. People who could help you count out your meds, make sure you were taking them on time, making sure that you had what you needed. Given that I had kids, I couldn't stay in the facility super long, so I had good family members and friends who came out to help me with them after I left the facility.

Zola's children are now eight years old. They don't remember much about their mom's battle with cancer, but they do remember how they felt when she was recovering.

They remember very vividly that they couldn't lie next to me, that they could've hurt me. They remember things I don't know why a five-year-old kid would remember, but they do.

That has translated in my life in that now, at eight years old, my twins aren't out of my bed yet. I mean, they start out in their own beds. But at some point during the night, they walk into my room and they crawl up under me because, for them, it's safety.

I don't think I'll ever know what it must've felt like for them to be told, at five years old, that they were going to hurt Mom if they snuggled with me. There is something psychological there, for a kid to believe that their hugs and love could potentially hurt their parents. So I think they carry a little bit of that now. I think that's part of why they need to be so close, because for a long time, them just being in my bed and laying close to me was associated with the thought of, "That's going to hurt Mom."

▪

There's the question of how long it takes for a scar to heal or stitches to dissolve. And then there's another aspect, which is, what does it take for you to have the energy to get through a day?

▪

THE COMEBACK

Since her bout with breast cancer, Zola has been thriving professionally. She joined producer Scott Budnick, who had spent several years raising money for a startup production company called One Community. They launched in 2018, with Zola serving as chief content officer. She and her team were creating films that, beyond entertainment value, carried social impact. Among them is *Just Mercy*, starring Michael B. Jordan as civil rights activist and attorney Bryan Stevenson. After a year helping get the company off the ground, Zola decided to take a step back.

I realized that my energy level hadn't come back to the same place that it was. The reading of twelve scripts a weekend and being out every night, before I got sick, I could do it with my eyes closed. All of a sudden, being at a film festival and watching six films a day and doing that for ten days straight, I just couldn't do it. I sat down with Scott and I told him that pretty candidly. And I talked to the board pretty candidly.

I said to them, "I want to figure out a way to do this, but I have to be able to do it at a pace that I can work with."

Among Zola's current projects is a film about Alice Johnson, a woman who was serving a life sentence for a first-time nonviolent drug offense, whose sentence was commuted by President Donald Trump following reality star Kim Kardashian West's efforts on her behalf. Zola is working on projects that matter to her, and doing it on her terms.

What's been great is that I've had the flexibility to be able to calibrate the ebb and flow of the projects. This is the first time that I've worked for my own company. I just said to myself, "I don't want to get sick again. I don't want to run myself down." I have to be able to do this at a pace that I can succeed. I knew that having fewer projects that I could do really well at was going to be the answer.

KATHY MATSUI

I think we are all placed on this earth to serve. And I feel
while I'm very lucky that I'm alive and I have a great family and friends and I work for a wonderful company, I have
an obligation to help others who might be in the same
boat as I was in, in the spring of 2001, who are totally lost
and may not have that infrastructure of support.

■ ■ ■

Kathy Matsui is vice chair of Goldman Sachs Japan, co-head of Macro
Research in Asia, and chief Japan equity strategist. She has been ranked
No. 1 in Japan Equity Strategy by *Institutional Investor* multiple times.
She was also named to *Bloomberg Markets* magazine's "50 Most Influen-
tial" list in 2014.

Her groundbreaking 1999 research on "womenomics" in Japan, a theory that female workforce participation would lead to economic growth,
reverberated throughout the country and indeed the world. It later became a pillar of Prime Minister Shinzo Abe's economic platform.

THE DIAGNOSIS

The year before she was diagnosed with breast cancer, Kathy was experiencing one of the best years of her life, both professionally and personally. She had just become the first female partner at Goldman Sachs
Japan, and she and her husband were celebrating the arrival of their
second child, a baby girl.

The year 2000 was the year that everything went right. The birth of my
second child, my #1 ranking, my partner promotion, and of course you feel
nothing could go wrong when everything goes wrong. Not even a year
after that, I was diagnosed. When I got the second confirmation diagnosis

that it was cancer, I said this to my colleagues: "You know what, this really is inconvenient. I'm just too busy to have cancer right now." Everybody laughs when I say that, but I really felt it.

You go from being completely in control and thinking that everything you do is in your power to, all of a sudden, it's out of your control almost completely. So it really was a major wake-up call and obviously super humbling. You find yourself thrown into this maze of doctors' offices and terminology.

Kathy had a family history of breast cancer, so she had long been scrupulous about her screenings, even at the age of thirty-six.

My mother [who lives in California, where she and Kathy's father ran a flower farm] had it, and both my grandmothers had it in Japan. So I knew I was at some degree of risk. I had done regular mammograms, and I was pregnant with my second child, so I didn't do X-rays but I did do my monthly self-exam. And I felt a lump and I thought, "Well that's strange." I had it biopsied in Japan, and they said it could be malignant. Of course, I said, "I'm sure it's not," and I had it re-biopsied in the States, and then it was confirmed.

I had already had a business trip to California scheduled, and I know nothing about the medical establishment in the States, but my younger brother happens to be a physician, and he actually specializes in oncology at Johns Hopkins. He helped secure me an appointment with a breast cancer specialist at UCSF, so I was able to get in whatever round of tests I needed and then get my results pretty quickly. So I'm very lucky—that was just the beginning.

There's no black and white in the whole treatment process. It's all so gray. So I wanted to get the best recommendations for how I should be treated, and it was all over the map. So my brother shepherded me through.

The next step was for Kathy to decide where to pursue her treatment.

I did check out options in Japan before making the decision to do everything in the States. They have cancer hospitals here, basically just for cancer patients. The treatment protocols, the drugs they use, that was all pretty much the same in terms of global standards. But what I felt was missing was two things: One was my language barrier. I'm fluent in Japanese in a business context, but I'm definitely not fluent in a medical context. So they're throwing out all these terms at me, and I could barely catch a fifth of what they were saying.

Second, and somewhat related to this, is just overall bedside manner. Everybody complains about in America how there's no universal health care. Well, the good thing about universal health care is that everybody gets access. The bad thing is that everybody gets access. So the amount of time a doctor can spend with you, even with a cancer situation, is pretty limited. That's not just with cancer; that's overall.

Kathy decided to have her surgery at home in California, where she recovered at her parents' house in the Monterey Bay area.

That kicked off a whole series of decisions I had to make about how my family's going to be taken care of and how my work's going to be taken care of. It was all just a super blur. I don't really remember all the details. I just remember I had these things I had to get done, and frankly I had no time to be emotional. I had to get back on a plane and book my surgical appointment and line up physicians for all the treatment that was going to take place.

The woman who ended up doing my surgery in California was my age. And she was so sympathetic, she'd say, "Whatever you need, call my cell phone, email me." She was just super understanding, and I felt that was what I needed.

If it was something not so serious, I probably would have done it in Japan. But in this situation, all the books say, all the advice says, you've got to be comfortable with the people taking care of you. And I just didn't feel that level of comfort here. That resulted, though, in separating my family. My husband was working here, my daughter was not even one year old. I eventually brought her over, so we were a split family for about eight months.

Kathy was putting together a medical team in the States, but would also be saying goodbye to her professional team in Tokyo for a while.

Although most of my colleagues are Japanese, and many are of course male, I didn't feel like it was uncomfortable to tell them. Of course, some of them reacted in shock and didn't quite know what to say, but it didn't cause me to refrain from telling people.

Telling my colleagues was like an item on my laundry list: "I've got to take tell my daughter's day care center, I've got to deal with my nanny who is going to help my husband and my son." I was just too busy. I told them I'd be connected, but they said, "We won't bother you if you don't want to be bothered." And I said, "It's fine. I can check in once in a while once my surgery is over and my chemo treatments are beginning, I'm going to have a lot of time on my hands, so I'll be in touch." But it was all pretty loose-ended.

In Japan, you just say you're on medical leave or you're just on leave, and the conversation ends there. Some people asked, "When is she going to be back?" And nobody knew when I was coming back. I had no idea when I was coming back. So you just sort of say, "I'm planning to be back, I don't know when that will be, but this will take at least half a year."

I didn't have a lot of lead time to prepare my team, but they had been working with me basically the entire time I had been at Goldman until that point. They knew the routine, they knew I wasn't going to be able to write reports for a long time, so they would have to cover and do whatever research and writing they could in my absence. The client-facing stuff in terms of meetings and marketing was obviously not going to happen, but to the extent they could write pieces and cover topical things that came up and still deal with client requests, they could definitely handle it.

Telling your colleagues is one thing, and then telling your clients is another thing. It wasn't as if I told all my clients, blasted out an email saying, "I've got cancer and I'll see you later." Those with whom I was close knew. Others, frankly, had no idea. They had heard that I had gotten sick and was going to be out of the market for a while. They weren't probing or asking difficult questions. But there were a couple in there who later on, their wives or they themselves were impacted by—it didn't have to be cancer. And having known what I had gone through, it was easier for them to open up about what they were going through or what their relatives were going through with me.

And in interviews with Japanese media, I wouldn't talk about it all the time, but in some cases I would talk about it. And that's also a very unusual thing, to be relatively high-profile and then talk about what you've gone through in terms of an illness.

Since she was a top executive at the Japan office, Kathy was expected to inform the senior leadership team herself. That included then-CEO Hank Paulson, who a few years later became U.S. Treasury Secretary. He just happened to be visiting the Tokyo office when Matsui was disclosing her news to the rest of her colleagues.

I had just made partner the previous year. Hank probably knew who I was because he has to call all the partners when they make partner. My colleague said, "Here's a time slot. Go in and speak with Hank. It will only be a few minutes—he's very busy—but it's best that you tell him yourself." And I thought, "OK. I'll try to think of a way to say it." So I stepped in the room, and he's a huge guy. Like football-size. With a very deep voice. We were in a very small meeting room with no windows. You could fit like four people, and he took up the space of half the room.

I said, "Hank, I just have something to tell you." I didn't make chitchat beforehand. I knew that he was really busy, so I just blurted it out. "I was just unfortunately diagnosed with cancer. I don't know how long I'm going to be away from work, but I really intend to come back and I'm sorry for the inconvenience."

And then he said two things: "Number one, don't worry at all. The firm will be waiting for you. Anything and everything you can do to get better, the firm's resources are all available for you if you need it." And then second, he said, "Just remember one thing: The best enemy of fear is love."

And I had held it together for that whole meeting, until he said those things. And then the faucet turned on. And thankfully he had to leave the room, so he couldn't see me in my puddle of tears.

He's a man of faith. And I thought that was such a moving thing to say. He said it with such conviction. And I said, "Wow. If this big guy, this very important guy at the firm, can say something like that, and say it with meaning, OK. I don't have to worry about work. I just need to take care of what I need to take care of, and the firm will wait for me."

I think for anybody going through something like this, to feel that the employers will be waiting for you is huge. And I don't think enough of that frankly happens in the world and here in Japan.

And when Hank said all the resources are at your disposal, he really meant it. We have—I didn't know this at the time—but we have an office in New York which is staffed with professional physicians and nurses. And because I'm a research analyst, my coping mechanism in the early months was just trying to figure out what the latest treatment protocols were, if there were any clinical trials that were just released. I just needed to get my hands on information. And so the nurses there, I bugged them to death to give me this document and that document. Not that I could understand what I was reading when I got the documents, but it just felt empowering to have this information.

THE BATTLE

When she was undergoing chemotherapy and radiation in the United States, Kathy had lots of time to think through some very heavy topics. She needed a sounding board, so she joined a local support group.

From the diagnosis onward I knew I was no longer "in control," that something else was dominating my life. It was affecting the way that I thought about myself, my future, my family's future. I was questioning whether I would come back to Japan, whether I would go back to work— my children were tiny at the time.

My parents live in a part of California which is close to a retirement community, so most of the women in these support groups were my mother's age. And when you would go around the table and introduce yourself and what your background is, I'd explain what I do, and it was like, I might as well have been a Martian from Mars. "You cannot go back to that way of life. That's just going to result in a recurrence"—they didn't say that, but you could tell by the faces and the comments that what they meant was, "Girl, you gotta change your life completely! Because this is not conducive to a healthy lifestyle."

I would explain my work life and work style, and having two small children and traveling a lot, late hours, conference calls, multiple times a week—it's kind of an unusual life. And so it was natural for somebody who was not accustomed to that kind of lifestyle to say, "You're still young, you have two small children; maybe you should, you know, pursue a hobby." Which is all done with very honest and well-meaning intent. It's not at all that I was offended by it. You start to question, "Maybe I should just become a stay-at-home mom." Which I seriously contemplated.

All these things would make you question the very core of what you believed until that day you received your diagnosis. I consulted with everybody I knew whose judgment I respected, from my best friend in elementary school to my college roommate. But nobody of course wanted to say, or was bold enough to say, "You should do this, you should do that." It was always, "You do what you think is right." Which of course is the right thing to say.

Kathy also had a community of other young survivors, thanks to her breast surgeon.

Before I went into the whole treatment process, she said, "Here's a list of women who have been at UCSF who are very similar in profile to you, who got diagnosed when they had little kids. They're willing to talk to any patients of mine." And first I thought, "Wow, that's really nice but no thank you." But then I started to feel compelled to call them up, and I called every one of those women. They were from very diverse backgrounds, but just to hear their stories, their decisions—you know, when they look back, would they have done anything differently? All these standard questions. But to be honest, just to speak to a human being who had gone through what I was going through who was alive and was striving, was so important for me at that time.

It was her late mother-in-law, a German physician, who really helped her gain clarity on how, and whether, she should change her life post-treatment.

I said in my broken German, "I don't really know what to do, whether I should go back to work." And she said, "Well, let me ask you one thing: How do you feel Sunday nights around 8 or 9 p.m.?" I said, "I feel totally exhausted, stressed out, and usually looking forward to Monday morning because I can go back to work and somebody else can deal with the kids." And she said, "Now take that sentiment and imagine that you're going to be the one at home, basically 24/7, with your children. And of course there are going to be lots of fun times, enjoyable times, but also it will come with all the stressful parts as well." And I thought to myself, "I don't know if I can take that."

It was this moment of, "Am I making a decision because I think it's right for the kids?" And she said, "Look. All I'm trying to say to you is if you are unhappy, for whatever reason, believe me, that unhappiness will ultimately project on your children. Whatever decision you come up with. Maybe you go back to work and you're unhappy. That will project on your children. Maybe you stay home, and you'll become unhappy. That will project on your children. Just think about that."

I thought, "Well, work is kind of routine. I know what to do and it gets my mind off the illness." When I'm at home, it was kind of a different story. I remembered, for maternity leave, it's kind of fun for the first few weeks and then it's kind of boring. So I just said, "OK, when you put it that way, maybe I should try to go back to work." And she said, "You don't have to go back and be the same 150 percent energy level as before. You tell people you are going to ease into it, and if it doesn't feel right, you say it doesn't feel right." And I always said to myself, "If it doesn't feel right, I can quit. I'll move on and do something else." With that attitude, I decided I would come back to Japan to work, and my husband and I would leave ourselves open to the idea that if we need to make an adjustment, we'll make it.

■

"You cannot go back to that way of life. That's just going to result in a recurrence"—they didn't say that, but you could tell by the faces.

■

THE COMEBACK

Kathy stayed true to her word and eased back into her high-powered job.

> I came in a little bit later than I used to and went home a little bit earlier than I used to. I definitely didn't accept business trip invitations right off the bat. I really just kind of needed time to transition back to work and back to Japan, so it took a while. Nobody pressured me, and it helped that people knew what I had gone through, so my managers were very sympathetic and my colleagues welcomed me with open arms. It was like coming back to my second home, because I had been at Goldman for over a decade.
>
> I came back and I had no hair. I had a wig so everyone could tell. It looked horrible, and you could tell it was a wig. But in the winter, it was really cold here, and I definitely needed something on my head because it was freezing outside. Yes, it makes people uncomfortable, but then again, how are you going to avoid that?

But Kathy knew that she had benefited from other women being open with her about their struggles. So she's tried to pay that forward.

> I think being open about it helped people gain access to me vis-a-vis their own challenges. All of a sudden, out of the blue, I'd get these emails or phone calls from colleagues, many who I don't know or don't interact with, saying, "I've been diagnosed," or "My wife's been diagnosed," or "This guy's been diagnosed with something totally different. But I would like to speak to you."
>
> I think oftentimes we look at people who are senior, and think, "Wow, they've just had this nonstop upward trajectory in their lives, professionally and personally." I don't know anybody who's successful in the world who's had a straight shot to success in either realm. And I think that opening up myself to talk about my experience, it makes me more vulnerable. And that vulnerability helps people access me and gives people a sense of, "Wow, she's a human being. She's gone through the things that normal human beings go through, and in whatever way, she survived. And I want to talk to somebody who survived."

I think we are all placed on this earth to serve. And I feel while I'm very lucky that I'm alive and I have great family and friends and I have a wonderful company I work for, I have an obligation also to help others who might be in the same boat as I was in in the spring of 2001 who are totally lost, who may not have that infrastructure of support.

MARY POWELL

I lead so much with my gut, and I think your gut is no
more than your brain's microprocessing unit.

■ ■ ■

Mary Powell served as CEO of Green Mountain Power, a Vermont energy utility, from 2008 to 2020. Under her leadership, GMP earned a
spot on *Fast Company*'s "Most Innovative Companies in the World" list
three years in a row (2017, 2018, 2019).

THE DIAGNOSIS

In 2015, at age fifty-four, Mary had already been undergoing routine
screenings for years because of a family history of breast cancer.

I always felt like there was something going on in my family history, not
just because my mom had had five distinct, unconnected cancers, but
because both of her sisters died of cancer. I also had, when I was young,
a female cousin, who was twenty-seven, die of breast cancer. Then I lost
another female cousin to cancer, and my sister had had breast cancer [in
2013]. I used to wonder, "Was there something in the water? Was there
something environmental?" Because my mom and her sister did not test
positive for the BRCA gene, which was THE gene everybody was talking
about and knew about. But I had been doing aggressive screenings always, as an adult woman, so I had had the mammograms, MRIs, and ultrasounds. They were using three different technologies to keep up with
me.

And then when my sister got breast cancer, she was the one who got
genetic testing, and it showed she had this gene, a [mutation on the] NBN
gene. There wasn't as much research on it yet. I decided just to get tested
to see if I had that same gene, so I did, and I had that NBN gene. And
while there wasn't, and may still not be, tons of data on the gene, there
was potential that it was tied to breast and colon cancer.

Sure enough, what do you think are the two cancers that have been predominant in my family? Breast cancer was universal throughout all of those women I talked about except for one, who was colon.

People always say I lead so much with my gut, and I think your gut is no more than your brain and your system's microprocessing unit. I think it's that little unit in there that processes all of your historical information and spits it out. So my gut was really strong that I should just take [my breasts] off.

Mary describes herself as "the opposite of a hypochondriac," so even though her gut was telling her to take preventative action, she found herself doing a cost-benefit analysis, as she would for a business decision.

There were all sorts of weird thoughts going through my head, like, "Well, I don't want to add to the health care problem we have as a country."

But then I thought, "If you do have cancer later, even if they catch it early and you have to go through chemo because of your family history, they're going to want to hit you hard with treatments, and that's going to be expensive, and you're going to be out of the workforce for maybe longer" because I'd seen a number of family members go through chemo and that's ugly.

I felt like, "Even if I end up just avoiding these mammograms and ultrasounds and MRIs for the rest of my life, maybe it'll offset the cost that way."

She decided to undergo a double mastectomy and reconstruction, choosing a doctor in New York City and staying with her brother nearby after surgery. But first Mary had to tell her daughter, Alex, about her genetic status and her decision.

It was emotional for me because she was in her freshman year at college, and I was nineteen when my mom was first diagnosed with cancer. So there was this funny "cycle of life" weight of emotions that was going on.

With Alex, my biggest concern was not wanting to frighten her. As a young woman, she had already been affected by breast cancer, because my mom had died of cancer before she was born, and she's always heard all these great stories about the grandma she never got to meet, so she's always known cancer has weighed heavily in our lives. I asked her if she wanted to go with me to any of the appointments in New York. We went together to the "fun appointment," to the reconstruction guy. And it was really cute because she wanted to go, and I had her help me pick out my new boobs. They have more types than I ever would have guessed. He brought out boxes and boxes. It was like choosing tiles for a floor! Telling me which ones are in my price range.

So I tried to just bring levity to it. She was there for the whole thing. And she pretty much adopted back then the approach that she's going to get tested at some point, and she's probably going to follow the same path as me at some point.

It was hard to tell her in some ways, but we faced a lot of different stuff as a family together, so in the scheme of things I just tried to include her as much as possible.

▪

> I had [my daughter Alex] help me pick out my new
> boobs. They have more types than I ever would have
> guessed.

▪

THE BATTLE

Alex was there for the surgery, which turned out to be one of the best decisions Mary had ever made.

I had just had all of those [tests]—MRI, ultrasound, and a mammogram— that were all completely clean. So after the mastectomy, they sent my tissue to pathology, and I'll never forget when the doctor walked in the door and said I was positive for breast cancer on both sides, in both breasts.

And I just cried, actually. I guess it was like crying of relief and crying of fear. I didn't know this when my body was screaming at me to have this surgery, which is what it really felt like, when I made the decision to do it.

And my doctor felt that because it was stage 0, I didn't need to do chemo.

As a CEO, Mary put transparency at the center of her leadership style, both for her customers and for her employees.

I've always been kind of annoyed with the word transparency. It's like, if you have to work at it, you don't have it. If you saw where we work, it looks like a colorful Costco. It's bright-colored offices with industrial ceilings, and I work at a standup desk right next to the linemen. I basically cut out all of the bureaucracy and the layers within the organization as part of the culture change. Our culture is about being one team and working together.

And so as a part of that, every Monday morning we start every week at 7 a.m., with a company-wide conference call that you don't have to dial into, but of the 500-plus people who work here, I would say about 400 do dial in every single week. We just talk about big picture things going on—safety and metrics—and it's usually no more than 20 minutes. And so as I was facing being out of the office for a period of time [recovering from the surgeries], and knowing that people were going to be wondering, and because we also talk a lot about health and safety as a company, it just felt like the obvious thing to me to tell them. So I told them about it before I went for the surgery.

The really hard call that took me by surprise was three weeks later. It was the Monday after I'd had that appointment where I found out I actually had stage 0 breast cancer, and I gave them that update. I got very choked up on that call, just sharing how grateful I was that I did the surgery.

Both calls created amazing connections throughout the company and had all sorts of unexpected positive impacts on other people's lives. There was a lineman who I didn't know, but he had breast cancer. We talk about it a lot with women, but as we all know, men can get it, too. I had more men share tears with me after my experience than probably any other time in my life.

For Mary, it was essential that she remained in touch with her colleagues while she was out of the office.

> There's times when you really want to unplug in life. And for me, after major surgery is not one of them. The emotional connectivity and strength I got from all the connections was worth its weight in gold. I think I was probably texting with people when I shouldn't have been, telling them, right after surgery, that I felt like I had a cement block on my chest with a tiger trapped underneath it. That's how I explained it, because it felt like a tiger was eating my chest.
>
> That part was painful, and I didn't want to take any kind of pain reliever aside from over-the-counter Tylenol, so staying plugged in was great for my emotional health. The team was amazing, so I felt like I could stay engaged, but I also felt like when I needed to just sleep, I could.
>
> A *New Yorker* magazine writer was writing an article about our company at the time and he was working on a deadline. He said, "Mary, I really need to interview you," and I said, "I just had a double mastectomy." Four or five days after the surgery I'm having this series of one-hour interviews, and the writer ended up doing a really incredible piece on the energy transformation that was happening at our company. But I have to say, I was sitting on pins and needles because I'm sure I wasn't at my intellectual best.

THE COMEBACK

Mary also wrote an op-ed for a Vermont newspaper, in which she called herself "the luckiest woman in Vermont."[6]

> After the op-ed, I was walking in downtown Burlington with my daughter, in the summer, probably four or five months after my surgeries, and this car pulled up, and this guy who was driving with a carful of other middle-aged guys shouted, "Hey you!" It was kind of out of nowhere. "Are you that…you're Mary Powell, you work at Green Mountain Power." And I thought, "Oh gosh, maybe it's a customer complaining—who knows." He made the guy driving the car stop, got out of the car, ran over, and said, "I just want to hug you. I want to thank you."

He told Mary that he, himself, had battled breast cancer.

Alex was right there, and he said, "Your mom, the fact that she had the courage to write about her experience, it was so powerful for so many of us who have dealt with these hard things and feel like we have to keep it quiet." It was just one of those unbelievable, life-affirming experiences of the power of love and the power of sharing ourselves and making ourselves vulnerable and the impact it has.

It has an impact no matter where you are in life, but when you are in a more public position, I think it has an incredibly strong impact. I don't know if folks think that we're supposed to be superhuman, but I think somehow, when you bare your humanity, it has very encouraging impacts on other people.

The other thing that was so surprising to me was how many women approached me and said, "Mary, I've been scared to even get a mammogram." And I'd encourage them, "No, you have to get a mammogram. The only thing to be afraid of is what you don't know, not what you might find out."

It still gives me chills on my neck. I had so many women say to me, "I think you've given me the courage to finally get a mammogram."

PART III

THE CHAMPIONS

When you play or coach a sport, you need to be in peak physical condition. For a competitor like Kikkan Randall, her body was everything: her sharpest tool, her deadliest weapon, and her closest partner. Decorated gymnastics coach Valorie Kondos Field wasn't competing alongside her gymnasts, but she still had to remain in top physical form to guide her athletes and demonstrate what she expected of them.

So when cancer appears, it can sometimes feel like a double betrayal. These champions worked their entire lives to preserve their bodies as their temples. How could they possibly become seriously sick?

But these athletic leaders turned to their teams for support. And that didn't just include their medical teams; their families and teammates also pitched in to help get them through their struggles. Kikkan's husband Jeff quit his job in order to focus on caring for her and their young son, while Valorie drew strength from her husband and the young women of the UCLA gymnastics squad.

But breast cancer also gave them an opportunity to step back, to understand on a deeper level that life isn't just about the numbers on a scoreboard. They've both reached the pinnacle of their chosen sports, but the taste of victory over breast cancer was a different sort of sweetness.

VALORIE KONDOS FIELD

Even though I have breast cancer and just got through a round of chemo, I still can feel the light that's inside of me. I'm not going to let cancer take that light away.

■ ■ ■

Valorie Kondos Field spent almost three decades as the head coach of the UCLA Bruins gymnastics team, leading them to seven national championships and 19 Pac-12 Conference championships, and helping shape the careers of numerous Olympians. She retired at the end of the 2019 season, and is the author of the book *Life is Short, Don't Wait to Dance*.

Valorie's success is made all the more fascinating when you consider that she knew nothing about gymnastics when she started. She was a dancer and had originally joined the UCLA Bruins as a choreographer for the gymnastics team. But her unique way of looking at gymnastics made her a brilliant head coach.

The whole concept of "winning" a performance is strange to me. But the gift was that because I didn't know anything, I had to ask a lot of questions. And I crafted my coaching style into asking questions. So when I had an athlete that was doing something well, or not well, I would say, "OK that was great. What did you do? What were you thinking? How did it feel?" Basically, they had to figure it out. And I didn't realize at the time that that was actually a really good teaching philosophy.

I think for coaches who are so proficient at their sport and their craft, it's so much more tedious to ask an athlete how they're feeling, and it's much easier just to dictate change—telling them "get your leg straight" instead of teaching them why it's beneficial for them to get their leg straight. My definition of a coach is somebody who motivates change. And in order to motivate someone, you have to get them invested into the reason why it's important for them to change. Not just tell them to. Now, we don't want compliant children. We want children that are excited about understanding why they should do something different. Even if it seems more monotonous or more tedious or has more steps to it, at the end of the day you're going to have a better result. Once you motivate them to really embrace the "why," then you can start talking about the "how," and you're teaching them versus dictating to them.

THE DIAGNOSIS

Valorie thrived on challenging the traditional way of doings things. So when she was diagnosed with stage I, HER2-positive breast cancer in 2015, she treated it no differently.

I had had regular mammograms once a year, but nobody in my family had breast cancer, so I really didn't worry about it. When I was diagnosed I immediately went into battle mode because I knew I was going to beat this thing; I was going to win. But I didn't know how I was going to win. And I thought about everything I had learned in coaching about resilience and perseverance, how the philosophy of failure recovery was so important because I knew I had setbacks but that I had to recover and move on.

When she first received the news, however, she described herself as "paralyzed from fear." That is, until she heard a voice speaking to her.

I heard God say, "Be anxious for nothing and be grateful for all things." I heard it twice, very clearly. I went home and I told my husband. And he said, "Yeah, it's from the Bible," and I looked it up.

"In everything give thanks; for this is the will of God in Christ Jesus for you." (1 Thessalonians 5:18)

"Be anxious for nothing, but in everything by prayer and supplication, with thanksgiving, let your requests be made known to God." (Philippians 4:6)

I was like, "OK wait a minute. What the heck is going on?" Here I have a potentially fatal disease, and I've been instructed by God to not be anxious but to be grateful. And then the next day I went to my oncologist, and she told me that, had I been diagnosed ten years prior, they would have had nothing for me [to treat it]. And I was like, "Whoa. OK. I get it." The way to not be anxious is through gratitude. I didn't *have* to get chemotherapy. I *got* to get chemotherapy.

Every single thing we do in life is a choice, starting with the thoughts that we feed and the thoughts that we starve. And I could choose whether to be scared, I could choose whether to have a pity party, I could choose to say "why me?" I could choose to think negatively. I could choose to feed those thought bubbles or I could choose to feed the thought bubble of "Whoa, I live at a time that has the chemotherapy that can kill the [cancerous] cells in my breast. Wow, this is going to be amazing. This is going to work."

THE BATTLE

Valorie referred to her chemotherapy sessions as her "chemo spa."

I didn't use that term flippantly, and I didn't say it to give me a false sense of contentment. I actually meant it. A spa is some place you go to get better. And my chemotherapy was like chemo spa.

Another thing a lot of people love about going to the spa is time spent alone.

If I was going to go and do my thing, I wanted it to be my time, my away time. I had so many of my friends, my husband, everybody saying, "Please, let me come sit with you." I'm like, "I don't want you to sit with me. It's my time! I don't want you there talking to me. It's *my* time."

Also, from the moment I get to work, my day is filled with people. I do not lack for a social life. And so I really covet and protect my alone time, and I enjoy it. I'm never lonely. That's how I get refueled. And had I allowed my friends and my husband to come sit with me in chemotherapy, it would have been simply because they wanted to. It would have fulfilled a need in them. And it wasn't about them. This was about me.

■

The way to not be anxious is through gratitude. I didn't

have to get chemotherapy. I *got* to get chemotherapy.

■

That doesn't mean that loved ones aren't part of the healing process, of course. Valorie relied on the support of her husband, Bobby, and her team—and vice versa.

My husband has a really strong faith, and if you have a strong faith, it's easier not to worry. He said to me, from the very beginning, "Anything I can do for you just let me know. But if I'm not overly worried it's because I know you're going to be fine." And that was, to me, really helpful. I wouldn't want somebody questioning how I'm feeling every day. I wanted someone who was going to be on the same page that I was, that I don't know what my year is going to entail, but I'm going to be fine.

[The breast cancer experience] made me more intentional with my relationship with God. I've always believed in God. But then when I heard "be anxious for nothing and grateful for all things" [having] never read the Bible, [I realized] this was a commandment and a gift from God, sharing with me how I was going to get through this year without being fearful and anxious. Ever since then I have understood that it's important to have goals and to set a North Star for your life and then set a plan and work the plan. But ultimately, it's really not in our hands. I feel like my hands are off the steering wheel, but whatever comes my way, each day I'm going to give my honest, best effort toward it with gratitude and appreciation.

I also told the team and my husband, "First of all, don't treat me like I'm sick. Sick is when you have the flu. I have some cancer cells in my breast that I need to figure out how to get rid of. But I'm not sick." And I told them, "Please, I will tell you when I'm tired. I will tell you when I need to take a break, I'll tell you if I need a hug. But please don't treat me like I'm sick."

When I went to the gym [after the diagnosis] and told my team, they started looking at my boobs, and that's when I got the revelation that I could actually give them the opportunity to feel what a malignant tumor feels like, because it didn't feel like a small round pea. It felt like a pulled muscle. And one by one, they came up and started feeling the side of my breast where the tumor was. I swear, there were sirens going off in my brain, thinking H.R. would come down and fire my ass for having student athletes feeling my boob. But at that moment it was too important. I thought, what a great science class for them to feel what a malignant tumor feels like in a living, breathing human being.

And it was great. It took some of the scariness out of it. One of them said, "From the minute you told me that you had cancer, this big bold-print idea of 'CANCER' [was] in my brain. And after we talked about it, Miss Val, and after I felt the tumor, it was like 'cancer' with a little 'c.' It wasn't as scary anymore."

I went to the gym every day. I think I missed one day. I just gave myself one personal day in a year. But [my gymnasts] were great. And if they did come up to me, they said, "Hey Miss Val, how you doing? Can I do anything for you?" It wasn't, remorseful and like, obsequious, like, "Oh, Miss Val, are you OK?" It was just like, "Hey Miss Val, can I get you a cup of tea or a cup of coffee or something?"

Just because she had a strong support system and positive attitude doesn't mean Valorie's experience with breast cancer was stress-free. She opted for a double mastectomy followed by reconstruction, and she had four surgeries before she felt comfortable with her new breasts.

It was right in the middle of our season. I had the implants put in and my nipples were facing out. So then I had a second [cosmetic] surgery, and they were massive. My assistant coaches kept saying, "You know what? Nobody can tell. Why don't you wait until our competition season's over?" And I was like, "No. I'm not waiting until our competition season's over. I want all of this done as soon as possible. I am not waiting."

After surgery, the doctors wanted me to stay home for a week. And I said, "No." I stayed home for three days, and I went in the gym on my fourth day. And I had the drains [from the surgery] still put in and I had a big black poncho. The girls wanted to come up and hug me, and I had to say, "No, no, no. No hugs."

As a top college sports coach, she had plenty of resources and people willing to do favors—but neither cancer, nor much of the health care industry, cares about that. She really wanted to participate in a new medical trial for her type of cancer that would likely prevent her from losing her hair, but she couldn't find an "in."

I didn't have the struggles that a lot of patients have, even trying to get an appointment, because of my position at UCLA. Every patient says that the unknown is actually worse than knowing, and wanting to be so proactive with your treatment and not being able to because of the system, I can't imagine what that feels like, how devastating that is.

I am a totally solution-based type of person. There's no obstacle too big. And so I said, "There's a study out there. Yes! I am going to figure out how to get on that study." But I couldn't do it.

I did not like not being in control of that. But I came back to my mantra of, "Don't be anxious about it." So I thought, "OK, I'm going to go through traditional chemotherapy. I may get sick and lose my hair. Let's try to do anything prophylactic that we can do." And one thing that my doctor said was that if I could afford acupuncture the day before chemo and the day after, it will really help. So I got set up with an acupuncturist. The cold caps [scalp cooling systems that look like big helmets] will help you not lose your hair. So I got the cold caps. And I was just ready. I thought, "All right. I can do this." And then the night before I was supposed to start, I got a call that I got randomly drawn and put into the study. And it's the only time during my entire experience that I cried. Of happiness.

And then it made me feel even better when I could get the cold caps to some patients that couldn't afford them.

And right at the end of her last treatment, she had almost an involuntary release of emotion.

I couldn't believe I was done. I couldn't believe I was alive. It was like, "I'm done. I can't have this needle in me any longer." You have to sit there for an observation period to make sure that you don't have a negative reaction. And I was like, "Trust me, I've had a full year of this. I'm not going to have a negative reaction. I'm fine. I'm done."

I think it was because for a full twelve months I had done a really good job of staying calm. Through the double mastectomy, through four different surgeries, to get the boobs right, through all of that. And it all just came to a head, after a full year of having to be calm.

THE COMEBACK

That episode goes to show that even someone as deliberately, studiously serene as Valorie was during this period of her life can't always be the master of her emotions. And that's normal. It's healthy. But after her treatment, her commitment to calm persisted and made her an even better coach.

My job as a head coach was to figure out how to win. And I thought that if I could bring a little anxiety to the situation, I would have heightened awareness of how to win. But because I had chosen to obey "be anxious for nothing," I went into the national championship that year not being anxious. I remember just being on a competition floor at nationals and looking at every single one of my student athletes and just being so grateful for them in my life. And after that meet, one of my students said, "Miss Val, I've never enjoyed a competition so much because you were so much fun, and you weren't stressed out. And it allowed me not to be stressed out."

And then I remember thinking, "Well, that makes total sense." Because I coach my athletes to not be stressed. I coach them on how not to be anxious. Why would I think that I'm helping the situation by being anxious? So that was a revelation. And then I just started asking people that are in really serious jobs, like surgeons, military people: When you're in battle, were there times where it's beneficial to you to be anxious? And they said, "Oh God, no. Because you're not aware. You cannot have that heightened awareness and intuition if it has to go through anxiety first. And the truth is that your brain can't think two opposing thoughts at the same time. So it can't be in a heightened state of anxiety AND calm and clear. You can't have clarity when you're in that state."

The biggest change [during that competition] was that I allowed myself to dance. I'm one of these people that when I hear music, I don't care if I'm in the grocery store or pumping gas in my car. If I hear music, I start tapping my foot and swaying back and forth and dancing. And I allowed myself to do that on the competition floor, which previously was blasphemous, because on the competition floor you're there for battle and to win. You're not there to have fun and dance. But maybe dancing, and then consequently encouraging my athletes to dance with me, put them in a better frame of mind to compete.

Just a few years later, in 2018, Valorie led her seventh Bruins gymnastics team to the NCAA championship.

We all go through tough times called life. And I remember one of my athletes saying, "You know, Miss Val, every time I ask you how you're doing, you say 'great.' You don't have to put on a false front for me. You can tell me that you're not feeling great." And I said, "No, but I am feeling great because even though I have breast cancer and just got through a round of chemo, I still can feel the light that's inside of me. I'm not going to let cancer take that light away." And regardless of what the hardships that we're all going to go through in life—because none of us are exempt from that—if you can find and fuel that light inside of you, it helps get through the tough times. And that doesn't mean I'm Yippie Skippy Cathy. It means that I'm calm and I'm not anxious. Even when I'm sad I still can feel my light. And not be anxious.

■

Maybe dancing, and then consequently encouraging

my athletes to dance with me, put them in a better

frame of mind to compete.

■

KIKKAN RANDALL

To me, the pink represents energy, enthusiasm, confidence that just anything that comes along, you can tackle.

■ ■ ■

Kikkan Randall is a five-time Olympian and was part of the women's cross-country ski team, which won gold at the 2018 Winter Olympics in PyeongChang, South Korea. She is also an ambassador for AKTIV Against Cancer and sits on the board of directors of Fast and Female, an organization that encourages young women to stay involved in sports.

Even if you don't follow cross-country skiing, you'd be able to pick Kikkan out of a bundled-up lineup because of the shock of pink in her hair, which she started rocking in 2005, in order to change the perception of the sport as the boring cousin of alpine skiing.

I felt like cross-country skiers were often dismissed as just disappearing off into the woods for hours and being boring and not being very good. So I started putting pink in my hair to show, "No, we're these New Wave skiers; what we do is exciting and fun. And I'm a girl, but I'm strong." And then I started skiing fast, so then it became a good luck charm. It became part of my identity, so I've had pink in my hair ever since.

Shortly before her diagnosis, Kikkan had capped off her career with Olympic gold, winning the team sprint freestyle competition along with partner Jessie Diggins.

When Jessie crossed the finish line, I looked at the scoreboard and I saw "Number One, United States" and realized that we didn't just get a medal, we won the gold medal. The emotion just overtook me immediately. I think I let out some big, ugly, awkward roar and then ran over and tackled Jessie. And it was a surreal moment as we got up off the snow and we went over to where our teammates had been cheering for us all night. And we just all soaked in this accomplishment together.

THE DIAGNOSIS

Just three months later, still floating on air from the gold medal win, a newly retired Kikkan was celebrating Mother's Day on a hike with her husband Jeff and their son, Breck. They had recently moved from Kikkan's native Alaska to Jeff's native Canada, where Jeff had found a new job.

I was so excited to have a day where I could be with my family and take a deep breath and think about where we were going from there. And it was getting ready for bed that night, literally coming off of Cloud Nine, that I just happened to brush past my right breast and feel something hard. My first reaction was, "Oh my gosh, it's been a month that I haven't been training, and I'm already feeling my rib cage. My muscles are disappearing."

And then I felt around a little bit more, and I thought, "Actually, that little hard spot's moving around. And it kind of feels like there's two of them." Then I said to my husband, "Check it out." From that moment on, I had this sinking feeling. And it bugged me that it was Sunday night, and I couldn't do anything about it until the next morning. Even though I felt in amazing shape, I just wanted to get it checked.

So the next day I went into the mammogram department at the local hospital, not really knowing any better, and they kindly told me I needed to be referred. I ended up at a walk-in clinic because we were in this small town in Canada. We didn't have a family doctor yet. I finally got in to see the doctor and show him the bumps, but he reassured me that I was young and healthy, and this was probably nothing. But, to his credit, he did say, "Well, let's just go ahead and do a mammogram and ultrasound just to rule anything out." So that took a couple of weeks to get on the schedule. Until the appointment, I was mostly able to put it out of my mind. Then I went in for the mammogram and ultrasound, and then whatever they saw on the ultrasound was concerning enough to order a biopsy.

Kikkan ran into a radiologist friend of hers who was able to get her in for a biopsy that day. He called a few days later with the results, while Kikkan was in Sweden for a wedding.

I was on the way to the wedding when he called me with the results, that the biopsy revealed that it was invasive ductal carcinoma—aggressive—and to try to enjoy the wedding while I was over there for a few days. But as soon as I get back, it's going to be time to jump into figuring out treatment, because it was going to be something that had to happen probably pretty quick.

I was actually in the car with one of my teammates who had just recently retired from skiing as well when I got the call that I had cancer. Then, as soon as I got to the location of the wedding, I called my husband and we talked about it. I think I did relax for the most part. I wasn't going to tell my friends who were getting married because it was their weekend. And I thought, "Look, I can't do anything about it right now. I'm here; if anything, it's a reminder of enjoying the moment you're in." And I think I did a pretty good job.

I was also probably just in shock, so I hadn't fully processed it yet. I had planned to stay in Sweden for a few extra days, but this was just weighing on my mind, so I actually bought a whole new plane ticket home. And the first morning after I arrived home, Breck came running up to me and jumped into my arms.

I think that was the first moment where, like, I broke down. Because all of sudden I was thinking, "Oh, my gosh, am I going to be around for him?"

But Kikkan quickly switched into athlete mode, zeroing in on her goals.

It was like, "OK, I need a plan, I need a team, let's get working on this." And right away, fertility was a big concern for me. The fertility treatment wasn't covered by my insurance, but I got connected with Seattle Reproductive Medicine, and I felt really good about working with them.

Kikkan did not yet have Canadian health insurance, but she still had coverage under the U.S. Olympic Committee's Elite Athlete Health

Insurance Program. So she decided to pursue U.S.-based treatment, beginning with fertility in Seattle, followed by chemotherapy in Alaska.

My choice was either I could go camp out in Seattle for three weeks and get the fertility medication directly from them, and then you have to go in every couple of days to get ultrasounds, your egg count, and stuff like that. But I knew I already was going to be spending a lot of time away from home when I started the treatment, so they were wonderful in working with me. We figured out that we could have the medications shipped to a small town in Washington that happens to be about 40 miles from where I live, north of the border, and kept on ice. I could drive down, I could pick it up. I could give myself the injections. And my friend, who's a radiologist, helped me set up the ultrasound at the local hospital. I did have to pay for those out of pocket, for the full price, but thankfully, it was the Canadian system so it wasn't as expensive as it probably would have been in the U.S. That bought me two or three weeks at home, and at that point I was still feeling so good. I could get out and do mountain bike rides and running, full tilt. I did find that giving myself the injections and ultrasounds worked great. Then, when it came time for us to harvest the eggs, I just went to Seattle. And then I went straight to Alaska, and within a week I started chemotherapy.

She and Jeff ended up creating five embryos, only one of which survived and was considered to not have a high risk of miscarriage. The embryo, which they nicknamed "Little Frosty," is in storage in Seattle. Then it was time to begin chemo.

Initially, when I found out with my insurance situation that I was going to need to get my treatment in the U.S. somewhere, I called up my gynecologist and I just said, "Hey, I got this diagnosis. Who would you recommend?" So she gave me a list of people to start looking into right away in Alaska. And I ended up finding out that one of the breast surgeons she recommended was actually part of the ski team that I raced for when I was sixteen.

She was someone I totally knew from ski functions, but I had no idea she was a breast surgeon. I thought, "Well, shoot, I want to go with her, because I knew her personality a little bit, but I also knew she would recognize me as where I'm coming from as an athlete, all the things I wanted to be able to get back to doing." Right away, that felt like the right fit. And then I knew one of the oncologists through some of the athletic events that I'd done in Anchorage. She came highly recommended, so I got linked up with her.

Over the course of that first week or two, we decided that we were going to do chemotherapy up front. That also bought me a bit more time, because initially it was gonna be like, "OK, we're doing a double mastectomy, reconstruction, all that," which is a big decision. And I felt at first that that was just what I had to do. And then it turned out that because I had chemotherapy in front, I got time to really weigh the options, learn more, think about it, and ultimately, I ended up going with a lumpectomy.

THE BATTLE

Fertility and breast cancer treatment alone are incredibly expensive, but when you add in all of the travel Kikkan was doing, the price went up exponentially. So they had to get creative.

It was definitely a little bit precarious there for a while. Coming off of my ski career, I was already unsure of how I was going to be making my income going forward, because in the past it had mostly revolved around me racing, and I wasn't gonna be doing that anymore. So then throw into the mix that I wasn't going to necessarily have control and be able to go out and do speaking engagements and participate in some of the things that I had planned to do.

But we were optimistic. We had some savings that could last over a few months if we needed to. And people definitely were there for us. We knew they had our back just in case things really went south. One of my sponsors did a GoFundMe campaign to raise money because insurance didn't cover the fertility and the back-and-forth of travel. And Jeff, having to be a single dad for a lot of the summer while I was in treatment, with day care costs and things, the community really rallied behind us and helped us with some funds to get through.

I was lucky in that a lot of people did offer to give me airline miles. I think we purchased a few tickets, but a lot of them people covered for me.

Kikkan brought Breck with her on her first trip to Alaska for treatment, and Jeff drove there separately in the Subaru Outback Kikkan had gotten in a sponsorship agreement, so that she had a car to drive while she was there.

> For the first round of chemotherapy, I actually came up to Anchorage about a week before it started. And I stayed there in Anchorage for the full first round, so that if I had any reactions or anything, I could come in for my weekly follow-up, and we could track how things went. So I committed to coming up to Anchorage for a month, and Jeff and Breck came up with me for the first week.

On the drive out, Jeff listened to a podcast called *How I Built It*, where entrepreneurs talk about the key moments in their lives that helped them reach success. Those conversations really stuck with Jeff, as he thought about how he could best help Kikkan during this heavy chapter in their lives. By the time he arrived in Alaska, he had an idea. After discussing it with Kikkan and with her blessing, Jeff quit his job to focus on being CEO of Kikkan Inc.

> **Jeff:** Kikkan was going to miss out on the opportunity to build off of the Olympics with the cancer diagnosis, knowing, especially in cross-country skiing, it's going to be a short window where you're going to get attention. Those athletes don't end up on late night TV being interviewed. I wanted to make sure that she was going to go through her cancer, recover, and get the chance to still benefit from all the years of hard work that would have been a struggle to do with the cancer. So I decided I would quit my job and take over running her stuff, or at least just get put on all the emails with her different partnerships, so that when she was struggling with the chemo or whatever, we weren't missing a week or two getting back to people. We stayed front of mind for them.
>
> It would have been one thing, just to end a career and then have some opportunities. But the gold medal is really something to build off of. It would open the door for people to learn more about her.
>
> She had a website. And when I got back and got to look at it, it was still a website of a hungry athlete who was trying to get people to follow along

on her journey. I looked up some other athletes with comparable results and just realized we needed to update it, so we contacted the company that had helped design it, and we did a revamp on it. And then, once we announced she had cancer, she went up 10,000 followers. She grew more on social media announcing she had cancer than winning the gold medal. So we realized we had to professionalize [her social media].

Jeff thought about how he and Kikkan could create something to help people connect with her and support her battle, both symbolically and financially.

She wore these tie-dyed colored running shoes to her appointments, and she called them her happy shoes because it lightened the mood in the room. And I realized, "OK, well, we can't create shoes. That's too much. But we could do socks!"

We had a platform and an opportunity to help other people that are going to go through cancer. The socks had the saying, "It's gonna be OK." I couldn't figure out something that would rhyme with Kikkan. "It's gonna be OK" was a hopeful message, and the K could be the signature "K" from her autograph. And then we donate two bucks from each pair of socks sold back to this cancer foundation, AKTIV Against Cancer [which advocates physical activity as an integral part of cancer treatment].

Jeff had been a stay-at-home dad for most of Breck's life up until that point, given Kikkan's chaotic schedule.

[When Kikkan was competing after Breck was born] there was no way for her to continue as an athlete without getting a nanny or something. We didn't really want to do that. And she was skiing well enough at that point that we could afford for me [to not work outside the home]. I actually worked in the winters. I worked on the World Cup [doing sales and mar-keting], plus she was racing November to March. And then we'd take the money I made doing that and pay for a family member to be with us on the World Cup tour, so from April 1 to the end of October, his first two years, I stayed at home with him. So I was already ready for that when the cancer part came around.

When this all happened, Breck was just over two years old. That was actually challenging because it was the first time he started to recognize that Kikkan wasn't around. For some reason, he just became super-aware. We were in a brand-new place. We were putting him in a day care for the first time in his life.

I was dropping him at day care because I was still working full-time when it first happened. I had to drop him at like 7:15 in the morning and pick him up at a quarter to 5:00 because I was working 7:30 to 4:30. So Mom's gone. And then I'm leaving him at a stranger's house. Maybe I was putting my own feelings onto him. I don't know what he was really aware of, but I didn't want him to feel like he was being abandoned. So I didn't fight making him sleep in his own bed. I enabled him for a couple weeks.

The day care lady was kind enough to give me a slightly extended day, so I would get home and then we would sit and have a popsicle on the front step as a make up for being gone all day.

Even when they were apart, Jeff supported Kikkan emotionally as best he could, helping her keep perspective when things got hard.

Kikkan doesn't like to show that she's hurting. If she tripped going down some stairs and broke her wrist, she would jump up right away and try to shake it off. Like, "No, no, let's keep running. I'm fine." So the days that she struggled with the chemo, I knew that she must be really hurting. Maybe "hurting" is not the right term. She didn't have pain, but she was uncomfortable. For sure there were some scary days. But we just had this talking point where we just said, "It could be worse."

She was so frustrated that she wasn't going to get the chance at the moment to have a second kid. And I was just like, "Hey, we gotta keep some perspective here. The news we have is that you get to stay around for the first kid we have. Let's not get ahead of ourselves. What do we have? We have a great little guy. And it sounds like you're going to get to be around to see him grow up. I think we need to focus on that."

While Jeff held things down on the home front, Kikkan was beginning her chemotherapy in Alaska.

Kikkan: For the whole three weeks between my first and second round of chemo, Jeff and Breck weren't there, but I was staying with my parents. They were there to take care of me. I rode my bike to my first treatment session. And I actually stopped at a local fitness club on the way. I knew going into the infusion that I felt good. So I thought, "You know what? I'm going to take advantage of the fact that I know I feel good right now. And then after that, we'll just have to see." So I did a hard workout and then got on my bike and made it to the hospital. And then that first infusion was seven hours. And I didn't spend a single second of that time alone. A bunch of my friends came, and they sat with me for that seven hours. My mom and my dad brought me lunch and chatted with the nurses. And through it all, that day I actually felt pretty good. I rode my bike home.

The next day I woke up and I could tell something was different. But overall, I still felt pretty good. We had decided that day that I would make my official announcement that I was going through it. So we sent off the message on Instagram, and within seconds, messages of support started coming in from all around the world. That whole first day was just managing all the support that was coming in. Media requests, flowers were arriving by the hour. It was just insane. I knew I was well supported as an athlete, but this took it to a completely new level. I was blown away. And then day two [after chemo], I think I still felt pretty good.

But then by day three, it started to hit. I just started to feel flu-ish and my GI system got thrown off. And that day I went wig shopping with a bunch of my high school friends. I had been warned that my hair would probably fall out sometime between three and six weeks. We were able to have a good time—trying on wigs was quite hilarious, actually. But I remember, sitting in that chair and putting the first one on, feeling like, "Whoa, this is real."

I'd already decided that I was going to make the commitment to stay active. I had told myself, "No matter what, I'm going to get out and I'm going to try to do something for ten minutes. And if I still feel crummy at the end of ten minutes, then I can always turn around and go back and rest." But more often than not, getting out there helped. That first week, I remember I was lying on the floor at my mom's condo, and I got a text message from a friend that they were going to go hiking. I just was starting to feel pretty bad, but I said, "You know what? I'm just going to go hike. I can just go with them for a little while. You know, maybe it'll be good to get outside." And I ended up hiking with them for four hours.

I remember I didn't feel great, but I wasn't thinking about how awful I was feeling. I was out there with them and talking. And I think I found out later that they were pretty nervous that I was out there for so long. But it was just so great.

And then within an hour or two of finishing that hike, I actually felt better. Then from that on through the rest of the three weeks, I went back to normal, and I thought, "Oh, well, this isn't going to be so bad; the first week will be tough and then I'll have two weeks that are pretty good until I do my next round." At the beginning of the third week, I did start to notice my hair falling out. I could just kind of pull it, and strands would come out. I had booked a speaking engagement for that week, and I just wanted my hair to hang in there for the speaking engagement. So I gave a talk to about twelve hundred people, and then I went straight from there to my hairdresser who had been doing my hair for ten years.

I said, "All right, let's do it." And she shaved my head.

Then I did my next infusion, and then the next day I flew home. My first day or two, I felt OK. And then by day three or four I started to feel rough. Plus, my son had just started day care, and he brought home a cold. I got it and I lost my voice for like ten days, and I felt just awful. And I couldn't kick it. I ultimately had to get on antibiotics. That was my realization that, "Whoa, I have to respect this because my immune system is not as strong as I'm used to. This can actually get dangerous." So when I traveled, I would wear a mask, and I would really make sure I was protecting my immunity the best that I could as I was traveling back and forth. For the third round, I just went up to Anchorage for thirty-six hours—I basically flew in the night before I got my infusion and then I flew home the next day.

I had told myself, "No matter what, I'm going to get out and I'm going to try to do something for ten minutes. And if I still feel crummy at the end of ten minutes, then I can always turn around and go back and rest."

As a world-class athlete, it was hard for Kikkan to reckon with being so physically fragile, even though she was used to being hyper-vigilant about her health.

I feel like I've had this theme throughout my life where I like to think I'm invincible.

When I got sick in that second round, that scared me a bit because I realized I'd been sick in the past when I was an athlete, and that was a bummer because maybe it meant I had to miss a race, which at the time felt like the end of the world. But in reality, that wasn't. This was serious.

In a way, being a skier did prepare me pretty well, because when we'd come into a major championship, you would be just doing everything you could to stay healthy. You're avoiding public places. You're washing your hands obsessively. You're wearing masks and, you know, telling your husband to go sleep in a different room if he has a sniffle. You just can't afford to catch it. So in a lot of ways, it was like back to being an athlete.

Following Kikkan's six rounds of chemotherapy, she had her lumpectomy and thirty-three sessions of radiation, which she completed in January 2019.

THE COMEBACK

Now, Kikkan spends a lot of her time doing motivational speaking engagements.

I like to share what I've learned through my journey as an Olympic athlete, through becoming a mom and returning to being at the top of my sport and then having gone through cancer and how there's been these similar themes that have helped me through these various challenges in my life. Those same themes can really be picked up by anybody to tackle whatever they face. And I love storytelling, planting that idea that we are stronger than we think if we take big, scary things and we break them down into small challenges, one step at a time. You'd really be amazed at what you can do.

And I just love to finish a talk and feel the energy in the room. I know how powerful role models have been for me. And I just hope to encourage young people out there, especially all the breast cancer survivors, that they can continue to get back to doing all the things they want to do.

Kikkan is definitely back to doing the things she wants to do. In addition to skiing regularly, she ran the 2019 New York City Marathon, completing it in less than three hours, which had been her goal. And her hair started growing, just in time for her to get her pink streaks back.

Every so often [before the diagnosis] I would get a question of whether or not the pink tied in with breast cancer. At the time, all I could say was, I participated in some events, I definitely support women who are going through it and staying active as a way to try to prevent it, but I didn't really have a personal connection, so it was just so ironic to find out three months after I won an Olympic gold medal [that] I have breast cancer when I have the pink in my hair. And it's also kind of ironic that through cancer, you lose your hair. So the one time in fifteen years I haven't had pink in my hair was when [I was] going through breast cancer treatment. To me, the pink represents energy, enthusiasm, confidence that just anything that comes along, you can tackle. And maybe it's fitting that it represents being a breast cancer survivor as well.

▪

We are stronger than we think if we take big, scary

things and we break them down into small challenges.

▪

PART IV

THE LEADERS

WOMEN WHO RUN for and serve in elected office have it hard enough. It's historically been a man's world, and in recent years, while women have made huge gains, they're still underrepresented in the halls of Congress and statehouses across the country.

And female candidates have to surmount huge political hurdles that their male counterparts hardly have to hop over. Among them is the outdated but nagging perception that women politicians won't be able to devote their full attention to public service if they are also raising a family. And women also have to address the flip side of that argument: that women who aren't married and/or mothers can't relate to the average voter.

Data backs the pesky staying power of those attitudes. A recent study in the *American Political Science Review* found that voters "reserve their highest reward for women who can both do the job of a politician and that of a wife and mother."[7] In other words, the authors write, "female candidates have to be superwomen, while male candidates enjoy the luxury of delegating family work to others."

Now add to that "superwoman" ideal a diagnosis of breast cancer.

The politicians in this chapter have all had to deal with that, either when they were running for office or serving. For some, breast cancer seeped into their campaigns. Then-gubernatorial candidate Heidi Heitkamp's opponent and his surrogates used her diagnosis against her. But when then-AG Christine Gregoire ran for governor in her home state, her battle with cancer ended up being a symbol of her resiliency. But the fact that these female leaders were going through something as universal as breast cancer meant they were able to reach all voters who had been touched by the disease in a unique and personal way. Putting aside politics, all of the women spotlighted in this chapter took advantage of their high profiles to perform that most basic public service: helping other people understand that they were not alone.

PAMELA CARTER

[Breast cancer] provided an opportunity as a leader to step out in the public domain and really talk to people throughout the state of Indiana. So we tried to make it as win-win a possibility as we could.

■ ■ ■

Pamela Carter was Indiana's attorney general from 1993 to 1997, becoming the first African American woman to serve as AG of any state. She then joined Cummins, a power equipment manufacturer, retiring as one of the company's top executives in 2015.

Pamela has battled breast cancer three times. Breast cancer might have been a tough opponent, but Pamela was not a woman to back down from a fight.

THE DIAGNOSIS

Just before her first diagnosis in 1994, she had been preparing for four Supreme Court cases, all of which Indiana won, and had just triumphed in the Mike Tyson sexual assault case, which resulted in his imprisonment.

My radiologist came in and said, "I'm worried." The X-ray showed a very suspicious-looking lump, so she took a biopsy of me that day. I was going to Washington, D.C., later on that evening, and I did go because I had a Congressional hearing that I was testifying for.

My radiologist had asked me whether I wanted to come back [to get the results]. I asked her to just tell me over the phone, so she ended up calling me after the hearing while I was in Washington. She said, "The biopsy came back positive. We're fairly certain that you have breast cancer and we need to move very quickly."

I didn't tell anyone at this point. I found a surgeon and an oncologist, and we met with the radiologist. They said, "Here's the path. You do have cancer, we think that it is two centimeters inside, and we need to do a lumpectomy. It doesn't look like you may have to lose the whole breast." So I thought it was doable.

About 48 hours before my surgery, they said, "OK, now do you have someone coming with you?" I said, "I haven't told anyone yet." They said, "Are you serious? You have to tell someone!" So I told my husband, Mike. It was a shock to him because his older sister, also named Pamela, died of leukemia. It was very emotionally wrenching. And that's the reason I didn't want to tell him. I was really trying to protect my family. It was a bad decision but I think with good intent.

I told him after my son's basketball game. We were both there; we had come from different jobs and we converged at the school. We were walking to the school parking lot to get in our separate cars after the game. And when I told him, it looked like somebody had hit him because, literally, his head went back. It was like an invisible strike. And that I will never forget. He was just stunned. But he was by my side completely and was the model of a supportive spouse throughout this process.

THE BATTLE

The doctors who performed her lumpectomy found that she had infiltrating ductal carcinoma, but they also found cancerous cells at the outer edge of the tissue that was removed.

They said, "Look, we're going to have to go in, and we're going to have to remove your breast." In the process of doing that, I went back for a couple more surgeries, and they also removed nine lymph nodes, five of which had cancer cells.

She hadn't told her two children about her diagnosis when she went in for her lumpectomy. But then someone spotted her going in for an appointment to prepare for her next surgery, the mastectomy, and leaked it to the media.

My children found out in a hurried way, which I didn't really want. I was trying to protect them from bad news, and I thought I could get through it without letting anyone know, which was naive.

The newspaper called me and said, "Look, we're going to put you on the front page of the Sunday edition, above the fold." And I said, "I haven't told my children or anyone." They said, "We're going with it." I was angry, but also resigned. It was similar to getting the cancer diagnosis. It was already here, so to go back and think other thoughts wasn't helpful for me. I was trying to think of what the next steps were. Once I found out the paper wasn't going to back off, I told them the truth, so at least they would know factually what happened, as opposed to gossip. I had to tell my kids 24 hours before it became completely public.

Mike and I sat down, and we told our children together. Our son, who's the oldest, was more stoic but very concerned. He asked a lot of questions and wanted to know what was going to happen. Later that evening we met with the surgeon and the oncologist. They took them through, showed them an artificial breast, so they could feel what the tumor would feel like. Our daughter, on the other hand, was completely emotional and dashed out of the house, running. I had to run out and catch her, and just hold her. It was tough for her. It was tough for both of them, but they handled it differently, emotionally. And the fact that they were having to process all of this both publicly and privately added to their burden.

Our daughter taught me a lot that day. She said, "You should have let me know." And that's why any time subsequent to that, I always made sure people knew. My mother and father were upset that I didn't tell them earlier. My sister—you know, we're a very close family. Beyond my nuclear family, my extended family were furious, and also protective because they know we're in this bubble, and this is all brand new. They wanted to help.

When [the story about Pamela] was published, it was front-page news, radio, TV, everything. On Monday, our children went to school. And our daughter, her class did government affairs on Monday, and I was the story. She only had one day to absorb the fact that her mother has cancer. I am, to this day, very, very proud of my family because I think they endured, not only a wrenching decision on a physical level, but their whole lives were exposed to the public domain well before we had adequately prepared ourselves emotionally and as a family. And they were completely resilient in so many ways.

Pamela was extremely close with her AG staff. Revealing her diagnosis to them had been excruciating.

It was one step removed from how wrenching it was to tell my family. I selected each and every one of the members of my staff, and it was one of the most diverse staffs in every conceivable way at the Office of the Attorney General. They are today and were then extraordinary people and lawyers. We were kind of a band of brothers and sisters, a little of a Camelot experience, and we came together to make a difference in our public service. On one hand they were just shocked and stunned and saddened, and on the other they were more emboldened and empowered to really make sure that our agendas for the people of the state of Indiana were achieved, successfully.

We had a big hundred million-dollar Medicaid lawsuit that we were focusing on. We had huge cases. During that time there was a big lawsuit that sued all members of the legislature, so we had their lawyers.

I tried to keep as much control of my body as I could, but in other areas, I let go a lot. And my staff, they stepped in with amazing swiftness.

During that time, I actually felt like there was a complete village around my family and me. To this day, that's one of the things that keeps me hopeful, to see that level of personal engagement, where people went way beyond what one would expect any human being to do for you.

Other times, people had already put me in the grave, so they would come to my house—and I'm sitting there—but they would talk to my husband Mike as if I'm not there, and they would whisper! There was also some real strange behavior where people would furtively look my way. I knew they were talking about me, whatever. People, when you're fighting cancer, engage with you in a strange way. So I'm more sensitive to, when people are undergoing similar or just difficult times, what not to do.

Following the media fiasco, she took steps to shield herself and her family.

When I went into the hospital [for the mastectomy], they didn't know which hospital I was going to, under an assumed name. And then after my surgery, they were actually going to each hospital to see where I was. We took my family out of the city to where I recovered. No one knew where we were. And I must say that during that time, Gov. Evan Bayh was amazing. He helped to find a place where we as a family could heal anonymously, which we did.

Two weeks after her mastectomy, she began her chemotherapy treatment.

I had six different treatment options every two weeks. The thing I remembered most was they were very unpleasant. My hair went away. Beyond that, you feel like you're pregnant, so that kind of hormonal feeling when you're pregnant remains with you.

And every subsequent chemotherapy session, I felt worse. I would get sick to my stomach on the third day after my chemotherapy, right on the dot. Just like giving birth. At a certain time, on the third day, boom! It would hit me, and it would stay with me for 24 hours.

I can remember closing my eyes in the fetal position, on my side, and everything hurt, including blinking my eyes. You could feel cell by cell. It's hard to describe it, but I would tell my mind to just kind of fight cell by cell.

But then there was something kind of magical, because in that 24th hour it would stop. And I remember getting up from the bed, and I would blink my eyes. I remember that because they no longer ached. And I would go outside, and the sunlight would hit my face. And I would feel the basic primal instincts of being alive.

I bounced back relatively quickly. But I was a petite person, and in addition to "chemo brain," where you forget things for a moment, I also got "chemo body." I blew up. It wasn't the steroids; they just called it "chemo body" at the time. I don't know that they knew what was happening. And then at some point, several years later, it just went away. But I did still work, except for a few days when it was really bad. Usually I knew that the third day after my chemotherapy I would take off. But more often than not I did work.

As hesitant as Pamela had been to have her breast cancer news leak while she was still in the early stages of fighting it, once it went public, she embraced her visibility.

I decided that, whether I lived or died, it would be a public process, transparent. So there were constant inquiries and opportunities for speaking. I spoke a lot anyway, as a statewide elected official. And women were empowered but also terrified. I had more women tell me that it was close enough that it felt very real to them. And also, being a public official was funny because there's no public space between you. Once I was filling my car with gas, and this guy, a complete stranger, came over and gave me a bear hug. I had never met him before or after. And he said, "I just know who you are and you have my prayers."

One of the things I did learn is that there are many medically under-served areas where women are inadequately diagnosed, they're not adequately treated. [Treatment is] very fragmented, it can be more expensive than it needs to be. I had a chance to have conversations with women constantly on that and move the ball a little bit. And that's when a lot of opportunities for bully pulpits joined with other bully pulpits, like Susan G. Komen and others. So we really joined forces and made some impact in those early days.

▪

Everything hurt, including blinking my eyes. You could
feel cell by cell. It's hard to describe it, but I would tell
my mind to just kind of fight cell by cell.

▪

A few years later, her cancer was in remission and her term as AG was coming to an end. She had to decide whether to run again, to seek higher office, as many people had been encouraging her to do, or to step away from public office altogether. She chose the latter.

I just thought, "My family has been through enough," even though my children in particular were saddened that I was stepping away from public office. I think, overall, they enjoyed it. My husband I think was delighted that I was coming out of office, because I think he was always worried about the stress and strain and the impact of that on my physicality and my future prognoses.

Right before she left office to re-enter the private sector, she was re-diagnosed with breast cancer. Even though they had removed the breast, some cancer cells had spread to her chest wall.

I felt a lump and I thought, "This couldn't be," because it was on the left side and I'd had the breast removed. So there was nothing there! I went to my OB-GYN actually, who did a fuller exam, and she said, "You've got a tumor here. I'm worried about that." And she sent me right back to my oncologist and breast surgeon. Indeed, it was a recurrence in my chest wall. That was in 1998.

This was well before laws prohibited insurance companies from jacking up rates for people with pre-existing conditions.

Part of that time [after leaving office] I was at a law firm, and then I went to a Fortune 500 company. And in both businesses, I had to let them know I was an active cancer patient. That was another opportunity for people to say, "No, I don't want to take a chance on you," but in both instances they said it was OK. I'm really a very lucky and blessed person for that to have happened.

Pamela began a radiation regimen.

I would go in early in the morning and get radiated, and then drive on down to Columbus, Indiana, from Indianapolis, which is where Cummins [the Fortune 500 company] is. I would take my kids to school and then go to Cummins. It felt like acts in a drama because I'd have different clothes on. I'd have gowns on for radiation, and then I'd put my suit on for work.

She moved with her family to Belgium and then to Tennessee, all the while climbing the corporate ladder.

> In all of those places I had fairly good care. I had brilliant care in Indiana. So when I went to get a mammogram, in maybe 2006 or '07, I didn't feel right. I remember there was an odd smell—a unique kind of antiseptic smell I had when I had cancer in the active form. I went and got mammograms, and they always have me come back because I've got dense tissue. They do ultrasounds, and they say "Oh you're fine."
>
> Finally, I said to my husband, "I am NOT fine! I just know it. And no one is confirming that." And I was going to the Mayo Clinic for my physical, so I decided to go and have them do a full everything for me, and the first thing they found was cancer, which I was not surprised about because I felt it. And I smelled it.

Sure enough, that doctor found some DCIS cells as well as stage II tumors. She had surgery and hormonal chemotherapy.

THE COMEBACK

Almost ten years after her third bout with breast cancer, Pamela remains healthy and happy, having retired in 2015 as Cummins' president of its distribution. She's also a grandmother three times over, so she's got her hands full. But she remains a dedicated advocate for women dealing with breast cancer—especially black women.

> The mortality rate among African American women from breast cancer is substantially higher, and it goes through the whole range of issues from living in medically underserved areas to having misdiagnoses, which happens a lot, particularly because there are not a lot of specialists around. I've seen a lot of women continuously go to physicians who are general practitioners who just don't know enough to be helpful, and it's distressing.
>
> To the point, all of my family go to the Mayo Clinic. My mother, my daughter, my youngest sister went to the Cleveland Clinic. But you also need comprehensive treatment. It's not just surgery or oncology or

radiology. It's a whole range. And usually women are not given a routine to help them through this process, so there's often a big gap that affects their health and recovery, and I think it accelerates negative outcomes.

These days, Pamela is still vigilant about her health, but is optimistic about the future.

I'm fine. I just came back from the Mayo Clinic. I just got tested from stem to stern, and I remain fine.

CHRISTINE GREGOIRE

I said to myself, "I'm not going to let cancer stop me
from doing what I need to do for the rest of my life." I
got right back on the horse and kept going.

■ ■ ■

Christine Gregoire served as governor of Washington State from 2004
to 2013. Prior to that she served three terms as the state's attorney general. In 2016 she served a term as the chair of the Fred Hutchinson
Cancer Center's board of trustees.

If Christine had decided not to run for governor, she might not have
detected her cancer as early as she did.

THE DIAGNOSIS

It was late August 2003 and Christine, who at the time was the state's
attorney general, had recently announced that she was running for governor. She decided that she should have a full checkup to make sure that,
if on the campaign trail she was ever asked whether she was healthy or
not, she could answer honestly. At age fifty-six, she was already getting
annual mammograms but decided to add another screening for good
measure.

I didn't think, when the campaign heated up, I'd have time to go in and
get one. I thought, "Well if somebody asks me that question, I need to be
able to give the answer that I'm fine." And it was actually quite fortunate,
because I caught it so early, and it was an aggressive form.

She had a biopsy following her mammogram. When she went in for the
results, the doctor insisted her husband be in the room. You might think
that would immediately raise red flags, but Christine was in denial.

I had had biopsies before, so I knew this wasn't normal. But I think I just assumed they were going to tell me something like, "Well, we're going to have to keep an eye on this."

We were standing looking at the X-rays, and the doc starts talking, and he just keeps going. He never uses the word cancer, but somehow I picked it up, and I couldn't hear anything he said after that. Finally, after some time went by, I said, "Wait a minute. Are you telling me that I have cancer?" And he said, "Yes." Then I said, "Well then, you've made a terrible mistake. You've got the wrong file. I'm perfectly healthy."

Early on I tuned him out because all I could think of was, "How could he be telling me I have cancer?" I could see his mouth moving, but I wasn't hearing him.

In an instant, Christine went from a state attorney general and gubernatorial candidate to all of those things, plus breast cancer patient.

I sat down and [the doc] said, "I can see how upset you are. What's upset you?" And I said, "What have I done to my daughters?" He was very reassuring and then asked, "So, have I addressed all your concerns?" To which I said, "Well, obviously I'm no longer a candidate for governor." And he said, "Can I ask you not to make that decision today?" I said, "That's fair enough." I just kind of put it out of my mind for a moment, because he scheduled surgery right away. It was a matter of days and I went in for the mastectomy.

Christine had an especially difficult time revealing her diagnosis to the two young women who mattered most to her.

This was the first time in my life that I had faced the fact that I wasn't going to live forever. I just never thought about dying. I never thought about being sick. I'd never been sick. And because of that, I probably tuned in a lot to the fear I thought my daughters would immediately have, that I was going to die and I'd be gone. So I struggled mightily. I waited until I got the biopsy back and made sure exactly what I had and what the future would bring. But before telling my daughters, we had just a few days. We didn't have much time.

My older daughter was down in Willamette, and we decided to tell her first. We thought it would be a good test for us, to see how she'd take it. No matter how much courage I had conjured up in my head to tell her, I [couldn't hold back the tears]. And, of course, she burst into tears. Then I said, "I'm crying just because I don't want to worry you. I'm confident, I feel good. Everything is going to be fine." I was disappointed that I teared up, but it was because I wanted her to not think she couldn't stay in school and keep up with what she was doing.

Then, we decided, "OK, we saw how well that went, and now we gotta tell the youngest one," who was still at home and still at school. With my second daughter, I was more composed than I was with the first daughter but still teary-eyed.

Me getting the message was so much [easier] than me having to tell the girls. I consider myself a pretty strong individual, but that was the biggest test. But I reached deep down to say, "You know my motto. There's nothing we can't do. I'm running for governor, I'm Attorney General, I can beat this, I'm going to get through with it, and you're going to be right there by my side." When I came home from the hospital, they were there and took care of me day and night for a couple days.

■

All I could think of was, "How could he be telling me
I have cancer?" I could see his mouth moving, but I
wasn't hearing him.

■

In addition to breaking the news to her daughters, Christine also had to figure out how to tell her staff.

When I told my executive committee, it was a sharp contrast to telling my daughters. I said, "Guys, I'm gonna be OK. It's gonna be fine. You're the leadership of this office, and you've gotta go out there and you've gotta be positive as you answer questions. So start asking me 50,000 questions—

any question, I don't care—so that you feel good about this." And they were great. And then I wrote a note that went to everybody in the office.

THE BATTLE

Christine had a mastectomy with immediate reconstruction in September 2003, a full year before Election Day, and she had to think hard about whether or not to continue her gubernatorial run. She also had to consider if and when to go public with her cancer fight.

> Part of the debate was, if I did announce it, would people think, "Well then she's out, she's not qualified," because of Heidi Heitkamp's story. I worried a lot about it. But then I thought, the potential to give people a wakeup call that they ought to get preventive care, at the end of the day, is more important. And anybody who thinks I'm not capable will watch me during this campaign and find out I am.

> Both my communications people at the AG's office and a campaign person that was a good friend of mine, we debated [whether to disclose the diagnosis] and decided that we would wait until after the surgery, at which time we would know more. Immediately after the surgery, the doctor confirmed there was no indication it had gone into the lymph glands; he had gotten it all by taking the breast. So that was considered positive news, and that's when we had the big debate about releasing it publicly. Could I—should I—not disclose? And I came to the personal belief that I was in such denial when they gave me the diagnosis, that I was probably not alone. There were probably many women who would be in denial that it could ever happen to them. If I was just forthright and honest, maybe I would influence people to get a regular exam—if they felt it could happen to their AG, maybe it could happen to them, and maybe we could turn what was a bad situation for me into something positive.

> And so we announced it and the response was, frankly, overwhelming. They would bring stacks of letters that I would get, and it would be typically someone who'd been diagnosed, who would say "You've now joined this sorority" and be very encouraging and supportive.

But she was not prepared for the intense fatigue she experienced for the first few weeks after her initial recovery, when she eased back to work.

I had the mastectomy and was in the process of recovering. I began to think, "I've got a lot on my plate, what am I going to do?" And again I decided, "I will begin doing work from home as AG. I'm obviously going to have to put the campaign on hold and think about it."

And about six, seven weeks [into recovery], I felt really tired, and, I remember, I went back in to see [the doc] to say, "Is this it? Am I for the rest of my life always going to be tired like this?" And he proceeded to tell me I was probably one of the most impatient patients he had seen. People make fun of me—every place I've gone, they call me the Energizer Bunny. And so to be that fatigued, I thought, "Oh my word. How am I going to live like this?" I thought it was forever.

I had not been back in the office and there was a retirement party and I'd been home for about two weeks. I thought to myself, "I'm going to that retirement. I'm going to pull myself to that retirement." Because when you're in a leadership role and people don't see you, they need assurance that you're fine. Sending a note that I'm fine, making a telephone call that I'm fine, doesn't hack it. So I went, and I got tired real quick and left early, but the time that I was there was exhilarating. And that's how I got back into it too quickly, too hard.

The doctor had warned that if you push yourself too hard, you'll really feel it and set yourself back. I remember a day in which one of my staff had come out to the house, and we were talking about an issue, and he went on the computer. I was describing what to do, and I was standing and walking back and forth, then suddenly I turned to him and I said, "We're done. I can't do another thing, I'm out. Done. Thanks for coming out." I realized much later, that was my hitting the wall. I had just pushed myself too hard, and my body gave me a wakeup call that there are limits to what we're going to tolerate. And so I tried to take a step back and then just ease into it a little bit more gradually than I had originally tried to do.

I started going in half days, and then half days become five hours, and then suddenly they become six hours and you're not paying attention to your commitment. So I had to watch myself. In fact, I remember going to my personal assistant and saying, "When I hit four hours, I need you to tell me, it's over. And don't let me say, 'Just give me another hour or give me another half hour.' Tell me. Remind me that I asked you to do this."

Then it was just like a flip of a switch at around eight weeks in, where I woke up one morning and I felt back to normal. And I said to myself, "I'm not going to let cancer stop me from doing what I need to do for the rest of my life." I got right back on the horse and kept going.

Christine also found guidance in the other members of her very exclusive club of state attorneys general who were also breast cancer survivors: Heidi Heitkamp and Janet Napolitano, who was Arizona's first female attorney general when she had a mastectomy in 2000. They both knew why she was calling before she even said the words.

I called them on the phone, and I said, "I need to talk to you privately, and you can't share what I'm going to share with anybody." One or both of them responded, "You have cancer." And I said, "Well, can you just answer my question first, do you promise?" And the answer was, "Yes, I do."

I talked to Janet and Heidi, and their experiences were not the same. Actually, that was helpful because then my experience was not the same, and I was OK with that. But Heidi's experience was so negative that it kinda stopped you in your tracks. Janet's was really very positive. She got through it and had public support. We talked about all the decisions you have to make. The choices were different in their cases but they helped me think it through, with the limited amount of time that I had to think all that through. And interestingly enough, I think we all three made different choices.

I'll be really candid with you: I got very down about the fatigue piece of it. So I kept asking them, "Is this what you went through?" And yes, they did. But recovery, I don't think, is the same for each of us. I've never heard anybody say they had the experience I did, where I just literally woke up one morning and thought to myself, "Oh my God, I think I'm back. I feel good, I'm going to be fine!"

To be a public official and to be diagnosed with breast cancer is different, and so to be able to listen to how they thought about it, how they worked their way through it, was really [helpful]. I've done my best to help others through it as well, because I think that sort of support is what we need to do for each other.

■

Then it was just like a flip of a switch at around eight weeks in, where I woke up one morning and I felt back to normal.

■

THE COMEBACK

Christine never imagined that her decision to go public would have so much impact on others.

I remember going to my first [Susan G. Komen] Race for the Cure as a survivor. I did the Race for the Cure before, but not in that capacity. They gave me this pink hat when I registered, and they said "survivors go over there," and I went over there and I was emotionally overwhelmed at the volume of people. I can't tell you how many women came up to me. And one very specific woman told me, "When I learned that you had breast cancer, I thought, 'If she had it, I could have it.'" She went in, she was stage IV, and she was a survivor. And she attributed that to my being open and honest about what I was going through, which led her to go in and have a mammogram.

It was at that moment that I said to myself, "Thank God that's what I did, if it could make a difference in that lady's life, how wonderful." And my last year in office, my husband had cancer of the colon. I said, "I'm going to ask you if we can share this publicly, because you may help someone who otherwise wouldn't be willing to help themselves." We sent a press release out, and the first call I got was Kathleen Sebelius, Secretary of Health [and] Human Services, who said, "Thank you, thank you. This honesty and openness are what people need to hear so they don't feel they're different or unique, and realize that preventive medicine is the key to saving your own life."

Her experience also helped her figure out how she wanted to continue making an impact after her two terms as governor. She became, for a time, the chairman of the board of directors at the Fred Hutchinson Cancer Research Center, or "The Hutch," a premier hub for the study of immunotherapy, or harnessing the power of the human immune system to cure cancer.

When I left office, everybody told me, don't accept any [obligations] for the first six months. I had lunch with a friend who asked me to go on the Hutch board. She said, "I agree with that advice, except for this."

I said, "You know what? This may be the biggest contribution I can give back in some small way to find cures." The detailed immunotherapy that Fred Hutchinson is doing may be the biggest breakthrough in cancer.

Besides that, I still have people who will call me and say, "You don't know this person but she's been diagnosed, she's a good friend of mine, sister of mine, would you be willing to make a call?"

The feedback I get is that when the governor calls, it inspires them, period. There's no question how much it's worth. But then we also have this very healthy, human conversation where then they realize it's not just the governor calling; it's a person who's been through it, and is telling you you're going to be OK, and that it's not going to be easy but that part of it is mental.

I am absolutely convinced that part of this is mental. Recovery is mental. And you've gotta be strong, you've gotta be positive, and you get yourself through it.

HEIDI HEITKAMP

Having cancer wasn't the hardest thing. It was seeing
my family go through having cancer.

■ ■ ■

Heidi Heitkamp has had a long, impressive career in business, politics, and law. She represented the Environmental Protection Agency and served as North Dakota's tax commissioner in the 1980s, served two terms as the state's attorney general in the 1990s, and was director of the North Dakota Gasification Company in the 2000s. Between 2013 and 2019 she represented North Dakota in the U.S. Senate.

When she received her breast cancer diagnosis in 2000, Heidi was running a tough gubernatorial campaign against Republican John Hoeven.

THE DIAGNOSIS

Like many women in this book, Heidi's breast cancer was improbable. Before she felt a lump in her arm, which ended up being swollen lymph nodes, all of her mammograms—including her most recent one seven months earlier—had come back clear. At first, her doctor assessed that the swelling was inconsistent with breast cancer and deemed it an infection.

He told me, "Take some antibiotics and then come back in like five weeks." And so I tried that for about a week and a half. And I'm bad at taking pills, so I wasn't taking the antibiotics. I also thought, "No, I need to find out what this is." And that's when we scheduled the biopsy.

It was creeping up on the campaign schedule. If I had waited to take a biopsy five weeks after I began a regimen of antibiotics, that would have put me in October [2000, a month before Election Day]. So I just said, "Look, let's just try and figure this out."

She went in for a frozen section procedure, where a surgeon removes a portion of the mass for rapid pathology.

I actually found out that I had cancer when I was coming out of the twilight from the biopsy.

One of the things that was unique was I didn't really have a discrete tumor, which is why the mammogram didn't pick it up. It was more like sheets of cancer cells. They said the pathology report showed a very aggressive form of cancer, which probably meant that I didn't have it that long.

The surgeon had looked at it and said, "We still can't say, based on the biopsy of the lymph node, whether this is breast cancer." It could have been an unknown primary tumor [which metastasized from elsewhere in the body]. So when we found out it was breast cancer, we were all pretty happy because that was much more treatable than an unknown primary.

Heidi's toughness was a strong refrain throughout her entire journey with breast cancer, beginning just the day after her biopsy.

The next morning, I did a parade, and ironically I ran into one of the recovery nurses in the parade. She just looked at me in shock, and I said, "I know you're sympathetic but we can't talk about it here." I kept working the parade, and then I went and sang at my nephew's wedding.

That weekend, I told my family because we were all together. [Heidi's husband] Darwin didn't want me to, because he's a physician and had a patient who had gone through exactly the same thing, who hadn't recovered. So he was freaked. He kept telling me, "This is way more serious than how you're acting." And finally I said, "Well, what do you want me to do?" He said, "You're in denial." I said, "So what?"

At this point, when she told her family—including her children, Nathan, age ten, and Ali, age fourteen—Heidi didn't actually know whether her cancer was breast, or some other kind. But then the news leaked.

There's a really horrible picture of me in the state capitol going to make the announcement that I had cancer with Darwin behind me. And Darwin looks like someone just took him out and just beat him. But we had to announce it before we knew what the cancer was.

I was AG at the time, so I just did it. It would have been news even if I hadn't been running for governor.

THE BATTLE

The notion of trying to answer questions about your sickness before you yourself have all of the answers would terrify most people. But for Heidi, it was business as usual.

> Politics is a mean business no matter what. So, you just kind of put one foot in front of the other. It's just politics.
>
> [Once her doctor was confident it was breast cancer], we scheduled the mastectomy, and about week after the surgery I was back on the campaign trail. And then I started chemotherapy. I think my first chemotherapy was the middle of October.

Before her mastectomy, Heidi had to have some difficult conversations with Nathan and Ali. She had to figure out the best way to talk about her mastectomy. But she also wanted her children's opinion on whether she should stay in the race.

> I remember, [the kids were] in the basement of our house watching TV. And I just came in and said, "This week I'm going to go in and I'm going to have surgery. They're going to remove the breast and then I'll have to take some medicine, but I think it'll be OK." And Nathan said, "Well, you're going to get a new one." And I said, "Well, no, I'm not. Because it would take too long." I knew that I needed radiation because of the kind of cancer it was, so we had already made the decision. Plus, I was in the middle of this campaign. There's no way I could do [breast] reconstruction because that was going to delay recovery and probably delay the radiation.
>
> Ali was fourteen, and I think it affected her more than it did Nathan. (Of course, it's hard to know with boys.) Ali was a competitive swimmer—she swam the 500. And she told me, "Getting out now would be like getting out of the pool in the middle of the race. Just finish it." She was saying, "Look, you got in this, you're almost done with this. Just finish the race, as long as you can do that and not delay treatment."

And finish the race is exactly what Heidi did. She had one chemotherapy treatment during the campaign, in mid-October, and one treatment after.

I think I was just running on adrenaline. It was the end of the campaign. The first chemotherapy was hard but not insurmountable. [She had a port implanted for the chemo], so you take blood thinners because they don't want the port clogging up, and I confused the anti-nausea medicine with the blood thinners. When Darwin found out, he's like, "Oh my God, if you get cut you'll probably bleed out!"

Unfortunately, Heidi's political opponents weren't above using her health struggle for their own gain. In a feature on Heidi in which a reporter followed her on the trail, *Self* magazine reported that a pollster knocked on a man's front door, asked who he was voting for; when he said Heidi, the pollster asked if he knew she was very sick, and then rattled off a series of side effects, including hair loss and weakness.

"And you're still going to support Heidi Heitkamp?" the pollster reportedly asked.

The Hoeven team denied having anything to do with dirty tricks like that, noting that they couldn't control every volunteer who went door-to-door for him. But one of Hoeven's top surrogates, outgoing Republican governor Ed Schafer seemed to have no qualms about bringing up Heitkamp's breast cancer as a campaign liability.

"I am concerned, really, in all honesty, that she has to go through chemotherapy and radiation," Schafer said in a radio interview in October. "I hope Heidi isn't going to get herself in a situation where physically it would be to her detriment to continue on this job."[8]

Schafer's wife Nancy filmed an ad that still sticks in Heidi's craw. Dressed in a silk pink skirt suit with a string of pearls, she speaks straight to the camera, saying that John Hoeven was the most qualified candidate for governor and that "he and [wife] Mikey are the best prepared to represent North Dakota to the world."

"We've learned that [the governorship is] really a team effort. You're the ambassadors for North Dakota," she says in the ad.

We called it "the pink suit ad."

And then [the late Fargo reporter] Kelly Stone got her ire up and went to Schafer and said, "What do you mean by that?" And he said, "Well, Nancy means that she's taken on all these things as First Lady, and she's afraid that they won't be followed through on, and that this is an important role, and [Heidi's] husband works full-time, so he won't have time." And then, Kelly asked him, "So, what things are those?"

And he said, "Well, like child immunizations and breast cancer." I'm not making this up. So when they asked me for comment, I said, "I'm not even going to respond to the breast cancer statement. But on immunizations, my husband can not only talk about them; he can give them!"

The Hoeven campaign had clearly made the decision that North Dakota was not ready for a First Family that looked like we did.

People would come up to her and urge her to get off the campaign trail.

People didn't know if I could be governor, like, "Well, she's a woman, and can she do this job?" And then you add in, "She's a mom. Can she do this and still raise her kids?" And then you put cancer on top of it. A lot of people wrote letters saying, "You should stay home and take care of yourself. We don't want you to risk your health any further." It wasn't mean-spirited in any way. It was protective.

But other women would come up to her and confide about their own breast cancer experience.

What was amazing to me was how confidential people held it. I would see someone coming at me, and I'd think, "She's a breast cancer survivor." These are women who never talked about it in their community, probably didn't even tell a lot of people in their family that they were going through it.

In my mother's generation, it was scarier to have cancer because the treatments weren't there. But there also was an element of "womanhood" to it.

But these women would lean in to me and say, "I'm a breast cancer survivor, too." And the older they were, the more they would whisper. And I'd say, "We're a hearty group!"

It was those furtive confessionals that partly inspired Heidi to film a campaign ad in which she addressed her breast cancer head-on.

"I'm not going to quit," she said in the commercial. "I believe in my future and the future of our state. In good times and bad, I'll never stop fighting for North Dakota."

Once we made the decision to stay in the race, then we needed to make a statement that we controlled, that was not being controlled by the media. And that's why that 60-second commercial was so important. To say, "Look, this happens to all of us."

By that time, I had heard from so many women. I hope that everybody appreciates this when they hear my story: Look, my husband is a physician. I never once had to worry about whether I was going to pay for health care. I had a supportive extended family. I had colleagues and friends who were going to support me. And I heard from so many women who didn't have that, who didn't have health insurance that was going to cover the total costs for single moms, or farm wives who didn't have health insurance, or didn't have the kind of support that I had, or were more isolated.

Some women choose a course of treatment that may not be as expensive or as intrusive so they can continue working. And that shouldn't be their priority. Their priority should be getting well—especially for women who are single moms and young and have a lot of life ahead of them.

So my story isn't a story of super grit compared to the stories that I heard over and over and over again.

■

People didn't know if I could be governor, like, "Well, she's a woman, and can she do this job?" And then you add in, "She's a mom. Can she do this and still raise her kids?" And then you put cancer on top of it.

■

And yet, Heidi's grit was still undeniable. While they were making the commercial, ad maker Mark Putnam had her do a few takes, and then she excused herself, going downstairs for fifteen or twenty minutes. The commercial team waited for her, she returned, and they resumed filming.

What he learned later was that during that pause, Heidi had been in her downstairs bathroom, vomiting because of the chemo. "And she didn't tell any of us," Putnam said. "She muscled on."

Heidi continued to muscle on, even after her hair started falling out.

> Lisa, my hairdresser who had gotten to be a good friend of mine, kept saying, "OK, I think we can wash it one more time." It was just glued on to my head on Election Day. Literally just hair sprayed on.
>
> I had a guy from the Democratic Governors' Association come out, and his job was to go behind me and take the hair that was falling off my jacket. How's that for the poor communications guy having to do that? And so the day after the election—literally that next morning—I went in and had my head shaved and got my wig.

Despite Heidi's positive attitude and popularity, her support in the polls slipped. Just after her diagnosis, she had a six-point lead in the race.[9] But by Election Day, she was ten points behind Hoeven.

> The life-changing moment for me wasn't getting cancer. It was losing the election. It was a really, really horrible moment. Probably the lowest ever in my life, because I had just lost an election and I got my head shaved.
>
> I think [the breast cancer] had an impact [on the outcome]. I'm not convinced I would have won even without it. A lot of people in North Dakota would say, "Oh she'd be governor if she hadn't gotten breast cancer." I will honestly tell you I don't think that's true. I think it was a bad year for Democrats. I would have had to get one out of every three George Bush votes. George Bush got a higher percentage in North Dakota than he did in Texas—I think we were third or fourth in the country—so Al Gore was very unpopular. It was a big Republican year.

THE COMEBACK

The publicity that accompanied Heidi's diagnosis had some positive widespread repercussions. There was a clear "Heidi Effect," in which her announcement prompted other North Dakota women to schedule mammograms.

"I'm getting women calling every day, saying, 'If Heidi Heitkamp can get it…then maybe it's time for me to get checked,'" the coordinator of a state women's health program was quoted as saying.[10] And while she lost her race, Heidi believes that her campaign helped her win the fight against her cancer.

> Everybody in North Dakota was praying for me, whether Democrat or Republican. And you can't tell me it didn't make a difference.

ANN M. VENEMAN ON THE POWER OF "GOING PUBLIC"

Most newly diagnosed breast cancer patients spend some time in the twilight of diagnosis figuring out how they're going to break the news to everyone, to "come out" as having breast cancer. Very few of them have the president of the United States Involved In the effort, but that's just what happened to Ann M. Veneman during her tenure as U.S. Secretary of Agriculture, in charge of policy for the nation's two million farms, the U.S. Forest Service, and numerous matters of international trade.

A year and a half into the job, Ann was diagnosed with DCIS, *ductal carcinoma in situ*, a non-invasive form of very early stage breast cancer. There was no lump. Rather, her mammogram picked up clusters of small calcium deposits lining the milk ducts of her breast, which can be an indicator of DCIS. With medical advancements in just the past few years, DCIS is now considered "stage 0" breast cancer.

As a member of the president's cabinet and the first (and still only) female Agriculture Secretary, Ann anticipated there would be a lot of questions about her health and whether she'd still be up to the job. Instead of a series of phone calls and meetings, she decided to write a letter to friends and colleagues to get the story out there quickly and consistently and in a way that did not raise alarm. The letter was also made available to the media:

September 18, 2002

Dear friends and colleagues:

At the end of August, I was diagnosed with a very early and treatable form of breast cancer. It is 98% curable and my doctors expect a complete recovery following treatment. I fully expect to perform the responsibilities of my position during treatment.

. . .

The month of October is National Breast Cancer Awareness Month, and particularly during this time, I cannot emphasize enough the importance of regular check-ups and mammograms. Early detection can make a significant difference in your life. There is a great deal of information available regarding breast cancer and I encourage you and your families to learn more about this important health issue.

While being diagnosed with cancer is not easy news to accept, I am grateful that it was not more serious and that with appropriate treatment, a full recovery is expected.

I am also very thankful for the support of my family, friends, and colleagues and appreciate your continued thoughts and prayers.

Sincerely,
Ann M. Veneman

As Ann was putting her letter together, she was told that President Bush was going to be holding an event for cancer research funding and she was asked if she would be willing to be a part of the event. The letter was released the same day the president touted her bravery in his speech:

Last month, Secretary of Agriculture Ann Veneman learned that she has breast cancer. This is one of the hardest things a woman can hear from her doctor, and one of the toughest challenges any family will face, including the White House family. Fortunately, Secretary Veneman's cancer was diagnosed at a very early and curable stage...I know I picked an extraordinary person when I named her to [serve as] the Secretary of Agriculture. I didn't realize I was going to pick a heroic figure as well, an example to many people to understand the need to get a mammogram; the need to take care of yourself; the need to screen early; the need to understand that we can stop cancer in its tracks if we all take wise moves. So Ann, thank you for your example.

Ann kept moving at full speed after her—and President Bush's— announcement. Shortly thereafter, she appeared on *Good Morning America*, talking about the importance of routine screenings. She had her lumpectomy surgery on a Friday so that she could recover over the weekend, and was back at work Monday.

I didn't miss a day of work. There were times when I was going through the radiation when I was quite exhausted. I had a couch in my office and on a few occasions I would just lie down for a half hour to rest. I would then resume my schedule for the remainder of the day.

Ann bonded with other female leaders in Washington who had been through the disease, including Supreme Court Justice Sandra Day O'Connor, who had been treated for a similar diagnosis several years before. Hundreds of well-wishers also sent her letters of gratitude and encouragement.

Following the announcement and the appearance on Good Morning America, *the outpouring of support was overwhelming. I received so many calls, emails, and letters from across the country and from around the world.*

Ann went on to have an illustrious career after her tenure at the Agriculture Department, serving as the executive director of UNICEF for five years and recognized on Forbes World's 100 Most Powerful Women list in 2009. But one of her most meaningful accomplishments was one she wasn't even aware of until well after it happened. A friend told Veneman that she had saved the life of an acquaintance who had seen her on *GMA*, talking about her breast cancer battle. She had been inspired to get a mammogram, and her breast cancer was detected early.

It was really quite heartwarming to know that maybe my experience helped someone else.

DEBBIE WASSERMAN SCHULTZ

I was stunned to learn that I, as an Ashkenazi Jewish
woman, was five times more likely to carry the BRCA
mutation than the rest of the population.

■ ■ ■

Rep. Debbie Wasserman Schultz has represented Florida's 23rd congressional district since 2005. She is also a former chair of the Democratic National Committee. By the time she was elected to Congress in 2004, Debbie had served in the Florida legislature for twelve years, long enough to have worked on numerous pieces of legislation related to breast cancer and women's health.

She was the lead sponsor on a bill to end the practice of so-called "drive-by mastectomies," in which insurance companies were denying women inpatient recovery services, forcing them to leave the hospital less than 24 hours after their surgeries. She was passionate about helping women dealing with breast cancer well before she realized she was one of them. But none of that prepared her for the shock of finding a lump in her breast at age forty.

THE DIAGNOSIS
In the fall of 2007, Debbie had her first mammogram.

It was a clean mammogram [but] it did indicate that I was at risk for calcifications. I didn't exactly know what that meant, but it was enough of a trigger for me to pay more attention to my breast health. A few months after that, I was doing a breast self-exam in the shower and felt this lump that had not been there before. It definitely felt weird and hard. You know how you played jacks as a little girl, the jacks have the ball on the tip of the spoke? It felt like that. And it turns out my tumor was less than half a centimeter, so it was really miraculous that I could feel it. I had my husband feel it, and he could feel it too. That was a Saturday, and I was home in South Florida.

I went straight to the doctor on Tuesday when I was back in Washington, and we made an appointment at Bethesda Naval Hospital [where lawmakers have access to specialists]. I ended up spending the entire day there because the clinical exam wasn't conclusive. They did a mammogram again, and that wasn't conclusive. They did an ultrasound, and that wasn't conclusive. They did an MRI, all in the same day.

At the end of the tests, the doctor gave Debbie a couple of options: she could have the tissue biopsied, or she could watch and wait to see what happened to the lump. Option #2 didn't appeal to her, so she decided to get a biopsy that day. When she was in recovery, her doctors expressed optimism that she was going to be fine and that everything "looked clean," although the sample clearly hadn't been sent back to pathology yet, where determinations about margins and how clean they are get made.

They definitely downplayed [the risk]. It was absolutely proposed as a viable option that I watch it and I wait. Which, because my cancer was stage IA, in the protocol that would have been perfectly fine. But it turned out I had a fairly aggressive form of breast cancer, so watching and waiting would have [resulted in me being] diagnosed at a later stage. Obviously, I had a tumor that the mammogram didn't detect. And they were very clear before my biopsy that it was probably not breast cancer. Because I was young. And that's statistically right.

I wasn't angry. Imagine the reality, if I didn't do a breast self-exam, if I hadn't gone in and had the biopsy. Not only did I have breast cancer, but I also have the breast cancer gene, and when they did my double mastectomy, they [found] DCIS in my other breast—which I didn't feel, nor did it show up anywhere. DCIS isn't as immediately life-threatening, but it can develop into invasive cancer.

I can't tell you how many young women I have spoken to who were dismissed, who were told to come back, who were told it was just a cyst, who were told, "Young women don't get breast cancer; don't worry about it."

Following the biopsy, she went on with her workweek. On Friday, she was back in her district.

I was at my district director's home for our office holiday party, and that's when my cell phone rang. It was the attending physician for the Congress [a position established in 1928 to provide medical care for lawmakers], and he said, "The pathology came back and you have breast cancer."

So when I hung up, it was like something was crushing me. I felt like an anvil had been dropped on my chest. I pulled aside my district director and my deputy chief of staff, who is one of my closest friends—in fact she was one of my caregivers—and I told them. I didn't tell anybody else that was there because my immediate reaction was, "Well, I gotta go figure this out before I decide how I'm going to deal with this."

And I didn't know anything at this point other than "I have breast cancer." I think the doctor said they thought they caught it early. So I think I had at least that much. But they didn't give me much more than that.

I had a four-year-old and twin nine-year-olds. That was the first thing that went through my head. I thought, "Holy crap. Am I going to live through this?" And of course, I knew the percentages, and I was being logical about it, thinking, "They said, 'We caught it early,' which means the chances are that I will likely survive," but at that point I didn't know what kind of treatment I had to have. They didn't know if there was lymph node involvement. Through passing breast cancer legislation as a Florida legislator, I knew enough about all the things I needed to worry about, none of which I had answers to at that moment.

I just said, "Well, all right. Tell me what I need to do." And then we set about doing it. I told my chief of staff, a very small circle of staff, and my husband, Steve, and my parents, my best friends who were going to help me in the aftermath. And that was it.

Steve is very logical. He's not emotional, but he's very supportive. We both deal with stuff like this in a similar way. We didn't freak out. I looked at the Internet once, and that was it. It made me freak out, and I was like, "OK, I'm never doing this again." I didn't do any research—no books, no self-help. I just told my doctors, "You tell me what I need to do, that is what I'm going to do." And, of course, I got second opinions. I was responsible about my health care, but I was not going to obsess. I mean, you could drown in it. And there was no way I was drowning in it.

One of the first things Debbie did following her diagnosis was discuss her family history of breast cancer, and her ethnic background, with her doctors. Debbie is Ashkenazi Jewish, whose descendants are from Eastern Europe. One in forty Ashkenazi women has a genetic mutation on her BRCA gene.[11]

I talked through my whole family tree. There was a lot of cancer—mostly lung cancer because we have a lot of smokers in my family, on both sides. Both my grandmothers died of lung cancer, and my aunt died of lung cancer when she was only thirty-two. And then I had two great aunts who had breast cancer, both in their forties. As soon as I said I had a great aunt who had breast cancer in her forties, and I'm an Ashkenazi Jew, and I had all this cancer on both sides of my family, the nurse educator said, "Because you're an Ashkenazi Jew and you've had breast cancer fairly young, you should go through genetic counseling and then make a decision about having the BRCA test." It made total sense. And it was more about the chances for recurrence because I had already had breast cancer.

When I walked into the attending physician's office at the Capitol for my appointment to get the [genetic test] results, it was one of those things where there were way too many people in the room for the results to be negative. I didn't even have to have them open the folder to show me because I knew. If it's good news, it's just going to be the one doctor, and that's it.

Debbie tested positive for the BRCA2 genetic mutation, which increases a woman's lifetime risk of breast cancer to 69%, ovarian cancer to 17%, and a recurrence of breast cancer in the opposite breast to 26%.[12]

After that, there was a total 180-degree shift on the recommended course of treatment for me, because initially, because I had such early stage cancer, they only were recommending a lumpectomy and radiation. And at that point, I would have possibly had to share my diagnosis [publicly].

But once they found out I had the gene, they said, "You have a decision to make. We recommend that you have a double mastectomy, but you could still have the lumpectomy and the radiation and you could just watch it. But given that you have the breast cancer gene, you're going to have to have an MRI every six months basically for the rest of your life." And I said, "OK, no. I am not walking around on eggshells waiting for the other shoe to drop for the rest of my life."

It wasn't even a question for me about having a double mastectomy. Besides, I didn't really have big boobs to begin with. I was an A cup, and I went to a C. I like to call my implants my "silver linings" because I was able to get a little more than God gave me.

Thank God I had nursed my kids. [My breasts] served me well, and I was sad to lose them, but I kissed them goodbye and told [the doctors] to take them.

When Debbie was diagnosed, her daughter Shelby was four years old, and her twins, Jake and Rebecca, were nine. Once she knew her cancer was very early stage and would not require intensive treatment, she decided that she would spare them the worry and not tell them about her diagnosis.

Anytime they'd heard about someone having cancer [at that time], it was associated with death. And I knew I had been diagnosed at an early stage and was more than likely to be OK, but I didn't want my kids to think or worry about, "One day is Mommy not going to be coming home?" Especially because I work out of town, traveling back and forth to Washington.

I didn't completely deceive my kids. What I did share with them was that Mommy is having surgery, and that I was having surgery to take care of something in my breast, and that I was going to be OK. But I didn't share them with them that it was cancer until after I was all done.

Once I finished with everything and told them, I still couldn't go into a whole lot of detail when they were that little. I talked to all three of them at the same time, and my little one, once she heard the words "but I'm OK now," ran out of the room and was skipping off and was fine. Because four-year-olds don't really know what cancer is.

My nine-year-olds, I had a longer conversation with, and I said to them that I had been through breast cancer for the past year or so and that I knew I was going to be OK but I didn't want to worry them. I was sharing it with them now because I was going to be publicly talking about it, so I wanted to make sure that they heard it from me. I talked with them later, when they were a little bit older, about the genetic mutation. They would hear me talk about it, though, when I gave speeches and things like that. That was a more gradual conversation, about their own risk.

■

[My breasts] served me well, and I was sad to lose them, but I kissed them goodbye and told [the doctors] to take them.

■

THE BATTLE

Part of why it was relatively easy for Debbie and Steve to keep the kids shielded until everything was over was because she spent most of the week in Washington, D.C.

I didn't miss any votes the whole time I was going through this. I had my double mastectomy in Washington, and I did it over the February recess, so I convalesced in my home in D.C. And I had my caregiving friends and family—they rotated in to take care of me during that whole period, and afterwards, when I went home to Florida.

I had a lot of different doctor appointments I had to go to through the course of the year in between the surgeries, particularly related to the tissue expanders for my reconstructive surgery. So I scheduled those at 7:30 in the morning. I was treated in Bethesda [Maryland, a D.C. suburb], so it was kind of a hike. But our caucus meetings were at 9 a.m., and I was usually able to make them.

Back home, Steve was with the kids all week.

My husband is the rock of my life. It was nice to have the confidence that he was able to hold the fort down, take care of the kids, answer questions that they might ask. Once I got home from the mastectomy, I couldn't lift things, and there were just a lot of limitations. And he was amazing. My husband is very low key and takes things in stride. He's not wound very tight. Also, we both trust doctors. We trusted in the team and the pathway that they laid out, which we decided I was going to pursue.

Unlike some other high-profile women, Debbie was lucky in that she could wait until she was ready to talk about her diagnosis and subsequent surgeries—and her new advocacy for women like her—publicly.

I had watched so many other high-profile people who had been through a serious illness be defined by that illness after they went public with it. And when you have cancer, it's so all-consuming, everything else in your life fades into the background. So what little you can control, you really savor. I didn't want cancer to define me. I didn't want a well-meaning reporter, every time they referenced me in a story, to write my name as, "Debbie Wasserman Schultz who's currently battling breast cancer." Because what I am is more than breast cancer.

I knew, when I was ready, I was going to use my position and profile to make a difference and fill a void. Everything fell into place when we started reaching out to breast cancer groups and it was almost unanimous that this was the void: Young women patients were really not a focus at all, of either the breast cancer advocacy community or of the research dollars that were allocated, and there was a huge deficiency in the awareness and the importance of young women paying attention to their breast health.

Because she was BRCA2 positive, Debbie also had to plan to get her ovaries removed—an oophorectomy—shortly after her mastectomy. Her surgical oncologist was intent on her having that surgery done as soon as possible.

> He could not get my ovaries out fast enough. He wanted to schedule my double mastectomy and my oophorectomy in the same three-week period. But I said no. He was concerned because the closer you get to fifty when you have the BRCA gene, the more likely you are to get ovarian cancer. And he wanted those out the furthest away from fifty that he could. I was done having kids, so that was fine. But thank God I listened to my own body and my own instincts, because I've never had more excruciating pain than my double mastectomy, besides childbearing.
>
> After my mastectomy, I had to stay in the hospital from Friday to Monday because it felt like I got run over by a truck. Even though nine days later I went to an event with Nancy Pelosi and was determined to move forward with my life, I couldn't imagine, another twelve days later, having surgery again. The oophorectomy was not very much, but you still go under. There was just no way I could have dealt with it physically.

The removal of Debbie's ovaries put her into what's known as surgical menopause.

> That was not easy but I probably didn't have the worst experience. I had hot flashes for about eight months. And then occasionally throughout the next several years. That was not fun. But the more important thing for me was that I had already had the children I planned to have, and I just kept thinking, "Thank God that I had my life play out the way it did." Because I know there are women that have to make that decision [to remove their ovaries] who maybe have not yet had kids or weren't married. And it's just so devastating and difficult.

Debbie's twins, Rebecca and Jake, are now twenty years old. Rebecca is taking her mom's advice to wait a few more years to get tested for BRCA.

> It's hanging over her head. Thankfully, she realizes that she can wait till her mid to late twenties before she has the test—but clearly not past that.

Hopefully she won't have the mutation, but she's already had that information far longer than I had it, and that's stressful. And then I've got to hold off my youngest daughter, because if her sister has this, then I'm sure that she'll feel a lot more pressure to want to know as well.

[Jake], he's a guy, and a college guy, and he is not thinking that way. But he knows that he's going to need to get tested before he has kids. His situation is different. He has to be slightly more aware if he does carry the gene for his own personal knowledge, because there are other types of cancer that you have an elevated risk for. But for him it'll be more about whether he would pass it onto his kids.

THE COMEBACK

Debbie is still a long way off from thinking about her legacy in Congress, but already knows that her work on breast cancer is among her proudest achievements.

The reason I always share that I was very involved in breast cancer advocacy long before I was a survivor is because I was quite familiar with a lot of the issues surrounding breast cancer. But I still didn't know, and was stunned to learn, that I, as an Ashkenazi Jewish woman, was much more likely to carry the BRCA2 or BRCA1 mutation than the rest of the population. I had no idea. And I realized that if I didn't know, then my gosh, how many other Ashkenazi Jewish women don't know that? Or African American women who don't know that their overall breast cancer risk is lower than white women, but that they are more likely to get triple-negative breast cancer?[13] And so they have to pay attention to their breast health for a different reason. And they also get diagnosed earlier, younger. So making sure that we fine-tune awareness and education and focus the communication in a more granular way is something I'm tremendously proud of.

THE EARLY ACT

The scarcity of resources didn't match the gravity of the statistics about breast cancer in young women. It may be rare, but at least one study shows it's actually more aggressive and potentially deadlier than breast cancer in older women.[14] According to the Centers for Disease Control, 11% of all new cases of breast cancer in the United States are found in women younger than forty-five years of age.[15] The Young Survivor Coalition says more than 250,000 women living with breast cancer in the United States today were diagnosed under the age of forty.[16]

Debbie spearheaded passage of the Education and Awareness Requires Learning Young (EARLY) Act, which was included in the Patient Protection and Affordable Care Act, the health care bill that became known as "Obamacare." The EARLY Act created a $9 million national education campaign targeted at young women to be aware of their risks, and a bucket of federal funding specifically for resources to help young women facing a diagnosis.

The other important element of the EARLY Act was educating health care providers to raise their sensitivity and their awareness about how young women present as breast cancer patients; educating them not to be as naturally dismissive of a young woman with a problem because breast cancer in young women is often diagnosed at a much later stage, which makes the treatment more involved, more expensive, and makes the mortality rate higher.[17]

We also have a grant program that provides funding to organizations that help young women deal with unique challenges when it comes to dealing with breast cancer. There's a huge difference between being diagnosed in your twenties, thirties, and forties, and your fifties, sixties, and seventies. I have heard terrible stories about doctors who didn't even suggest to young women that they preserve their fertility before they go through chemotherapy. Women were becoming sterile and unable to have their own children—at least with their own DNA. Young women have questions about dating. What date do you tell the guy that you're seeing that you had a double mastectomy? That's a kind of awkward conversation. My mom is in her seventies. If she had breast cancer right now, that's the last thing that she would have to think about. What do you do about nursing?

We have nearly 40 million dollars now appropriated for those buckets of education and awareness and additional money that has been appropriated to fund grant programs for organizations that help young women deal with the unique challenges that we face when we're dealing with breast cancer.

But the bill didn't get passed without a debate. Some organizations, including the National Breast Cancer Coalition, opposed the EARLY Act because they argued that the federal government should focus its efforts on a cure, not prevention. They were also concerned that the bill's passage might result in more women getting unnecessary screenings and biopsies. "The bill is addressed to a population of women in whom breast cancer is rare, and presumes we know what to tell these women about prevention, risk reduction and early detection. We do not," the NBCC wrote in a statement.

My argument at the time was, "What you're suggesting is that we write off women who are going to get breast cancer—25,000 women a year between 40 and 50 years old—and just say it's OK to let them die because we need to concentrate the research dollars on a larger percentage of women that get breast cancer, and that we need to not scare women into having biopsies that turn out to be benign, which would give the best news you could possibly ever get. I don't know any woman that's ever had a biopsy that came back benign that was upset that they had the biopsy.

They did, however, have some support in the scientific community and some still argue today. That's why there's still a battle over whether women between 40 and 50 should have a mammogram and why the U.S. Preventative Services Task Force *recommends that women don't need a mammogram between 40 and 50 and that it's only in consultation with their doctor.* *

One program the EARLY Act funds is called "Bring Your Brave," which shares stories of survivors and previvors under the age of forty-five, produces educational videos to address the sorts of concerns that young survivors have, and finds innovative ways to reach young women through pop culture.

For example, a character on the TV show *The Bold Type* found out she had a BRCA mutation, and on the night the episode aired, social media accounts for the CDC and for the show's producers shared resources for viewers to learn more. They did a similar social media campaign during an episode of *Grey's Anatomy* when the mother of character Dr. Maggie Pierce was diagnosed with inflammatory breast cancer, a rare form which causes the breast to swell and redden.

Kelly McCreary, the actress who plays Dr. Pierce, tweeted some facts about breast cancer and a link to the CDC's website, such as, "Most women who get inflammatory #BreastCancer have dense breast tissue, which makes it harder to find #cancer with a mammogram." She tweeted this with the hashtag #MaggiesMom to connect it back to the episode.

---

* As of January 2016, USPSTF guidelines recommend biennial screening mammography for women aged 50 to 74 years and say that for women younger than 50, "the decision to start screening mammography . . . should be an individual one. Women who place a higher value on the potential benefit than the potential harms may choose to begin biennial screening between the ages of 40 and 49 years."[18]

PART V

THE COMMUNICATORS

ONE OF THE maxims that journalists adhere to is to never make yourself the story. Keep the spotlight on the people whose stories need telling, whether it's about political corruption, personal triumph, or communal suffering. But sometimes, journalists can't help but recognize that their own story is worth telling.

As mainly broadcast reporters, the women in this section are all very publicly visible, so when they were going through their diagnoses, it was hard for viewers not to have questions. Some of them were able to report all the way through their cancer battles. Others took time away from their all-consuming jobs.

Some, like former *Good Morning America* host Joan Lunden, decided to guide their viewers through their sickness. Others, such as CNN correspondent Athena Jones, opted to wait, to "bury the lede" and not tell anyone outside their immediate circle until after they were feeling better, even when their viewers began to suspect that something was amiss.

But each has used her own story to help others with theirs.

JENNIFER GRIFFIN

Engage your kids. Let them be a part of it because they're going to know that something's going on. And it's a growth experience for families. It's a way for your children to learn empathy, and to learn that life isn't fair, and life is tough, and you can grit and get through it.

■ ■ ■

Jennifer Griffin is a FOX News national security correspondent. She joined FOX in 1997 as a Moscow correspondent and later moved to their Jerusalem bureau. She's also traveled extensively through Iraq and Afghanistan with various members of the Joint Chiefs of Staff.

Jennifer and her husband Greg were adventure-seekers well before Jerusalem. They met in South Africa in 1989 at the first legal African National Congress rally, shortly before Nelson Mandela was released from prison. Greg was the AP news editor there, and Jennifer was traveling during a year's sabbatical from Harvard University. They were married in Islamabad, Pakistan, when Greg was the AP bureau chief in Islamabad and Jennifer worked as a freelance journalist. They honeymooned in Kabul, Afghanistan. They spent Thanksgivings in the region hunting their own turkeys. They were both reporting in Moscow, Russia, when Jennifer was hired as a FOX News correspondent, six months after the network first went on the air.

Jennifer had spent her first two pregnancies living, basically, in a war zone. She was the network's reporter based in Jerusalem during the Second Intifada, a five-year period of heightened violence between Israelis and Palestinians. She had cut both maternity leaves short so that she could get back to covering the tumultuous history unfolding right in front of her.

While nursing, she would pump between interviews with Hamas leaders in the Gaza Strip, bringing bags full of expressed milk through checkpoints back to the Israeli side of the border. A few years later, she joined her FOX News coworkers on a harrowing search for two of their kidnapped colleagues, Steve Centanni and Olaf Wiig, meeting with militia leaders in dark alleys trying to negotiate their release (they were returned after two weeks). And on a personal note, her father had passed away just days before her younger daughter was born.

So when Jennifer found out she was pregnant with her third child, shortly after she and Greg decided to move back to the United States so she could become FOX's Pentagon correspondent, she was ready for a relaxing third pregnancy. She bought what felt like the ultimate indulgence for a war correspondent—a cozy rocking chair—and prepared for a period of nesting and post-natal bliss.

Unfortunately, breast cancer had other plans.

THE DIAGNOSIS

Jennifer had a family history of breast cancer: Her mom had it, and her great-grandmother had died of breast cancer at age thirty-five.

I started screening quite early—a little earlier than what they recommend. I probably was in my late thirties when I had my first mammogram in Israel. And in Israel, because there is a lot of breast cancer, it was easy to do. I had had at least one mammogram in Israel before we moved back to the States, so I thought I was being really on top of the preventive screening.

I was also under the mistaken impression that I had done everything right in terms of breast health. When I was pregnant, I figured, "Well, I'm safe." I had had my mammogram a year and a half prior, and I thought, "I'm pregnant so I don't have to worry about this right now."

That's why, as I was nursing my son—he was six months old—and I felt a lump, I just assumed it was mastitis. It was really hard, and it was in my right breast. My breasts were engorged because I had been nursing, so I didn't think anything of it, but as I started to wean him, it was quite obvious that I had a hard lump there. My husband noticed it, and I thought, "Ugh, I'll just go get it checked." I went to my OB-GYN, and he sent me to a radiologist. Breast cancer was the last thing in the world that I thought could happen, and I thought I had been on top of it. But what I later learned is that during the pregnancy, hormonal changes caused by pregnancy can actually promote the growth of cancer cells, so you actually do need to be extremely aware of breast health during pregnancy.

Jennifer credits her doctor for taking the concerns about her breasts seriously enough, when he could have simply advised her to wait out her body's postpartum changes. But as it turned out, she was diagnosed with stage III, triple-negative breast cancer, meaning the cancer cells were not growing in response to hormones or the HER2 protein, the most common triggers.

My OB-GYN was on top of it, probably because his wife had had breast cancer, but he also was quite amazed at how quickly something had appeared because he had checked my breasts during the pregnancy. I feel that my life was saved because we were quick once we realized what the lump was. I received the call on September 28, which was a Monday, that my biopsy results had come back, and that was Yom Kippur. I remember my doctors were both Jewish, and I thought, "Who's calling me on Yom Kippur?"

I was in the shower. My sister was here helping me with my son because I had gone back to work. She came in and told me that there was a doctor on the line. I thought I was headed to the Pentagon that morning for work. My radiologist actually told me over the phone that I had cancer. I don't know if he told me it was triple-negative or he just told me the tumor size [9 centimeters].

As a war reporter, Jennifer was used to receiving a piece of news that required her to snap into action.

It was as though I had been called to head off to Iraq. I think I was still in my robe. I put on my journalism hat and started researching and calling people—anybody I knew in the cancer world. [The neighbor of] a friend of my half-brother's mother was the top breast surgeon at Georgetown Hospital, so we started with her. I started research online, I didn't trust anyone.

Triple-negative, I learned, was newly named, and [in 2009] there wasn't a great prognosis. Now, I'd say we are learning more about triple-negative and that maybe it can be a better prognosis if you treat it in a certain way. All of my friends from high school and college immediately got on conference calls and divided up the research and ways in which to help the non-medical point of view. We did nutrition and exercise research. It was very clear, early on, that triple-negative responded to a very clean diet, vegan diet, and 45 minutes of exercise a day. I'm extremely Type A and I like to control things, so I started controlling everything that was in my power to control.

Within a couple of days, I had seen two sets of doctors and had two very different recommendations in terms of either starting chemo first or starting surgery first. One set of doctors wanted to go straight to surgery. I got in to see a team at a different hospital, however, and they were doing something that now a lot of people are doing, but at the time it was somewhat unusual, which was pre-operative chemo [neoadjuvant] to see whether the tumor responded. So we literally just watched, over a couple months and seventeen rounds of chemo, as the tumor melted away.

THE BATTLE

Once Jennifer decided on the preoperative chemo route, her doctor, who was on the cutting edge of treatment for triple-negative cancer, also improvised when it came to the chemo protocol itself. In addition to the recommended three-drug chemo, known as "AC-T" (Adriamycin and Cytoxan plus Taxol), she added carboplatin, a colon cancer drug which had been studied for its efficacy in fighting triple-negative breast cancer. Carboplatin is now a much more regular component of a triple-negative regimen, but it wasn't at the time.

It was a hard protocol, but I threw the kitchen sink at this cancer, and I had doctors who knew that I was serious about it.

Obviously, though, I was not all business up front. It was an emotional roller coaster. I had a friend from college take family photos of me with the children and with my mom before I shaved my hair. We posed on the couch—the same couch where we told our daughters, Annalise and Amelia, who were eight and six at the time. Annalise had had a soccer game that morning and was in her little soccer uniform. We brought them home, and

Greg and I sat down and said to them that I was going to start treatment and that I was going to lose my hair. Their jaws dropped. I said, "but just like Hannah Montana we're going to go and get the coolest wigs," and we just fixated on getting lots of different fun, rock star wigs. I ended up getting some funky wigs that were all different lengths depending on my mood.

And then friends flew in from all over the country when I shaved my hair. My six-year-old daughter was my partner in crime of videotaping me. [FOX News colleague] Greta [Van Susteren] brought me a video camera, and in fact she called me one of the first nights after I was diagnosed and had me on her show to talk about something else, because she knew that I needed to keep putting one foot in front of the other.

In eight years, we haven't looked back on those videos that Amelia shot. I don't think the girls realize how many videos we have from that period. It is almost like a documentary. It was extremely helpful, I think, for my daughter Amelia. My older daughter Annalise had a little trouble wanting to engage in it. She was just a little more scared of me when I was bald, but the six-year-old was just so close to me and always there with the camera.

We literally just watched, over a couple months

and seventeen rounds of chemo,

as the tumor melted away.

The professional challenges and personal danger that women at FOX News have endured have been well reported—something Jennifer is acutely aware of. But in her experience, her bosses, including the late Roger Ailes, who left FOX following numerous allegations of sexual harassment, were generous beyond what was required of them.

Roger ran FOX like a general, and if any of his people were in trouble, you knew that he was going to send in the cavalry. It was a complicated place from that point of view, because we all had such loyalty to him, in many ways. Since then, we've learned that some of our colleagues were really treated very badly, and there was an undercurrent of sexual harassment going on, but many of us—most of us, I would say—were unaware of that and were actually the beneficiaries of a great deal of kindness. And so it's hard to reconcile the two versions of FOX that are out there.

But from the point of view of a worker and somebody who, when you hit bad times or wanted to feel like an institution had your back, there was no better place to work. One colleague who himself had battled cancer called me because he knew what it was like to be diagnosed. He said, "What do you need?" And I was sort of getting a little weepy, and I said, "I need to be with my kids." That message got to Roger, and Roger sent a message immediately through [former executive] Bill Shine [who resigned from FOX in 2017 amid the harassment scandal]. Bill called me and he said, "You stay with your family, take care of your family. All we care is that you get well." And they kept me at full salary [for a year].

With that said, this author is aware that not all FOX News employees received this level of care and concern during a medical leave. But no one can deny that Jennifer had a completely positive experience. Even when she was on leave, Jennifer was focused on getting the story out there, and began a blog to keep her friends and family updated on her health.

I would be sitting at my dining room table at midnight, after everyone was asleep. I was jacked up on steroids from the chemo treatment and wired beyond belief. And I just wrote. It was so therapeutic.

10/6/09: Everyone says I must learn to visualize during this period. Some say think of Pacmen eating the bad cells. I prefer something a bit more militaristic. I'm the Commander in Chief. Al Qaeda cells have taken over parts of my body and I have signed the Execute Order and sent in the Navy Seals with a shoot to kill order. That works for me better than butterflies carrying off the tumors.

Sometimes people are opposed to the warrior-like rhetoric that is accompanied with fighting cancer. However, I found it worked. It doesn't mean that those who died from cancer didn't fight. It just means we've got a ways to go in terms of doing our research, in terms of our environment. There are carcinogens everywhere, and we have failed in terms of our ability to prevent cancer.

> **10/28/09:** First, my friend Jim sends me a pack of "Bald Guyz". Who knew there were special wipes to keep your bald pate feeling squeaky clean and fresh and who knew how itchy and sweaty a bald head can get? And now I know why Santa wore a kerchief because it is bloody drafty at night when you don't have any hair! Thanks, Jim, for letting me in on the inside track—now that I am an honorary member. I may never go back. Now that I know the benefits. Wash and go has taken on a whole new meaning. And I must say—it's a bit sexy!

Following her chemotherapy, Jennifer had a double mastectomy with reconstructive surgery. Then she had six-and-a-half weeks of radiation.

> **5/4/10:** [For radiation] I put on those two hospital gowns. The first one that opens in the back and the second one to cover me modestly so that the first one covers me modestly. I lost my modesty long ago—after two Al Qaeda tumors took my body hostage for 6 months and I began showing EVERYONE my breasts. They suddenly weren't breasts. They were the scene of a crime and became war zones. And I was proud to show anyone who cared to ask after we deforested and then rebuilt them. They've been through a lot. I don't really feel like hiding them.

She also wrote about how she overhauled her diet and exercise, including living by the mantra, "Cancer Hates Cabbage."

1/26/10: Many of you know I have become a huge fan of Pilates since starting chemo. I knew that ballet dancers and those on the Upper West Side seeking to look like Gwyneth Paltrow and Uma Thurman did Pilates, but I had no idea how it could literally save your life. Joseph Pilates, a German, came up with the philosophy to overcome his childhood rickets and developed it for hospital patients, not ballerinas. All of the machines are based on "hospital beds"... the springs, the position of lying down and doing these controlled movements that strengthen your core and boost your immune system. The unique way of breathing can literally increase the oxygen flow and raise your white blood cell count. I am using the controlled strengthening of every tiny muscle I never knew I had in my upper body, chest and arms to prepare for my double mastectomy. I am increasing the range of motion in my arms so that I will hopefully avoid lymphedema*—a common side effect of breast surgery after lymph nodes are taken out. But more importantly Joseph Pilates who was placed in an internment camp when he was in England during World War I (he was German, remember) taught the other prisoners mat Pilates—and those who did the exercises with him survived the outbreak of pandemic influenza. Those who didn't, well, didn't.

She also wrote of the hard days, like when she suffered a "psychological setback" after learning her doctor was going to extend her chemotherapy sessions past the original number. She found solace in rap music.

11/22/09: I reached back about 8 years to an old Eminem riff that had the necessary driving beat to drag me back to reality and drag my running shoes out the door

---

* Lymphedema occurs when excess fluids collected in tissue cause swelling. Radiation can cause the formation of scar tissue that narrows the remaining lymph vessels and nodes, which can interfere with blood flow.

and down Mass Ave. when the anxiety started to build and the tightness in my throat left me gasping for a little more breath. I downloaded "Lose Yourself" from iTunes and had a new mantra—a slightly angry one at that. "You have one shot—do not lose your chance to blow—this opportunity comes once in a lifetime..." Over and over it played as I punched my way down Mass Ave. tears rolling down my face. Angry that I had to waste another minute on this damn disease.

THE COMEBACK

Jennifer was in close touch with her friends, but the blog was also a way for her to unload her thoughts and emotions—unfiltered and uninterrupted. It has also been a great resource in the years since her battle, when she can't remember certain details.

This is the good news. You start to forget. It's like pregnancy. You start to forget your cancer story, which is good because when you live it and you know every little detail, you become like an oncologist where you know every scientific term for everything that's going through your body because you obsessively research it.

But that doesn't mean she's forgotten the profound, positive effect the whole year had on her family.

It was a very traumatic year, of which I still have emotional scars, but also, when I think back to the kindness and the fellowship and the community that came around me, it shaped my family. It shaped my girls. My daughters are college-aged now. Their teachers, throughout their lives, have recognized in them there's a light that comes from knowing how you can lose everything in a minute. Whenever they hear that somebody has either lost a parent or are going through something similar, they are the first to reach out. And unfortunately, it's happening more and more but I must say, that year shaped our family. In a good way.

Jennifer's blog was not just there to help her. She intended for it to be a resource to others. With that in mind, here's a post she wrote on January 17, 2010. It's a letter she wrote to a newly diagnosed friend with triple-negative breast cancer, but it might as well be an open letter to anyone diagnosed at any stage.

1/17/10:

Dear ****,

Your fear and your anxiety are totally normal. Being in shock at first is totally normal. So you do need a friend/ partner who can accompany you to every appointment and hear what the doctors are saying because it is hard for the patient to be little more than a deer in the headlights when you hear the big "C". . . It's easy when we are in shock to just go with what the doctors say but in fact this is the most crucial time. So be confident, be strong but as Ronald Reagan said: "trust but verify." I trust no one and I double check everything. Again, I don't want to create more stress for you, but I want to empower you to feel 100 percent confident with your course—so these next days are crucial before you start.

Here are some tips for handling chemo—take them for what they are worth (toss them out if you think they sound too kooky) but I find in this situation where you have very little control that nutrition, food and exercise are extremely helpful in handling the chemo—so here goes:

1) Get your teeth cleaned before you start because you can't get them cleaned during chemo and you tend to get mouth sores—you can minimize these by brushing your teeth 3–5 times a day and rinsing with a mild mouthwash—I use a mild dry toothpaste and mouthwash called Biotene (baking soda and saltwater gargles work, as well.)

2) Get your wigs now—find a really cute fun one or two and go with your girlfriends before you start losing your hair. Have fun with it—no one in Hollywood wears their own hair—they are ALL wigs—I am a redhead right now and never was before and love it. The typical chemo drugs cause your hair to fall out on day 14–17—shave it off before it starts falling out—it's much more empowering that way—invite your girlfriends to do it with you. Plan to have lunch somewhere fun afterwards. Embrace it. Bald is very powerful but remember to get a hat—a fuzzy fleece one— because bald is also breezy and you will catch drafts that you didn't even know existed. You need to sleep in the fuzzy hat all the time. I like to wear cute knit hats over the wigs because they look a little less wiggy and a little more young. (Let your friends throw a hat party for you—like a baby shower but with hats.)

3) Get some nice body lotion and lip balm because the chemo dries out your skin (on the flip side chemo is better than botox and takes all the toxins out of your skin and suddenly your face is as smooth as a baby's butt.)

4) Get some powder bronzer so that when your face looks pale and drawn and a little green from the drugs you can throw on a little extra bronzer powder and blush and feel that you don't "look like a cancer patient." There is a reason that the American Cancer Society has what is called the "Look Good, Feel Better" campaign because if you get up each morning and shower and put on your blush and your wig, you literally feel better. It is so easy to start the downward spiral into feeling sorry for yourself. There's a great title of a book: "Why I wore lipstick to my mastectomy..." My husband Greg once asked me why I was getting so dolled up? "After all," he said. "We were just going to chemo...." I told him that was exactly why I was

putting on lipstick and a bright scarf and great earrings. It's your body armor. Don't go out without it. Every time I have, I have regretted it.

5) Get some clothes that are your "chemo uniform". I went to Max Mara and got comfy leggings, long cozy sleek sweaters, furry boots (like Uggs)—cashmere everything. Anything to make you feel cozy and sporty. All easy to throw on—so you just reach in your closet and grab your uniform— taking all the stress out of what to wear.

6) Order from Amazon immediately two cookbooks by Rebecca Katz (a San Francisco chef) "The Cancer Fighting Kitchen" and "One Bite At a Time" and tell your friends about them so they can cook healthy things for you that help with the chemo side effects and not bring you donuts and cakes to make you feel better. . . . The drugs and the steroids can cause havoc to your metabolism so it's best to try to find a reasonable but pretty strict eating regime to give your body and immune system the strength it needs to fight and bounce back. Your mouth will feel like Chernobyl pretty quickly and your taste buds die so there are tricks in Rebecca Katz's books to make food still taste appealing and to stimulate your appetite so you can stay strong. Certain foods definitely boost your immune system.

7) I immediately eliminated all processed foods, all white sugar and nearly all dairy (Triple Negative responds well to a VERY low fat diet—to be a vegan is ideal, but you will find that when you get anemic during the chemo you may have to bend the rules a bit on meat—at least that is what I have found and was tucking into some veal shank for the marrow at midnight last night). Also a low glycemic diet is very good for Triple Negative because there is some research that shows that Triple Negative may have something to do with insulin levels.

8) I drink only water, bubbly water and green tea (don't want the sugars in the other drinks.) I put lemon in and on everything—it cuts through the chemical taste and you need 3 quarts of water a day to wash the chemicals through your system—staying hydrated also keeps you from being nauseated. They recommend 3–6 mugs of green tea a day to get maximum benefit from the anti-oxidants in the tea. Start eating all organic. Check out Jane Plant (British geologist's book) on how she survived breast cancer by giving up dairy.

9) Don't touch any milk, eggs, or meat that have any hormones in them. I still eat eggs and fish—but only wild caught fish—salmon and white fish—don't want the swordfish and other things that are higher up the food chain because they have a lot of mercury.

10) Eat a lot of cabbage—"Cancer Hates Cabbage!" (Chapter 10) When you are eating this clean detoxed diet filled with Super Foods then you are going to be as strong as you can be to counter the tsunami like effects of the weekly, biweekly or triweekly chemo treatments. It's like girding yourself to take each wave head on—like body surfing. And even those days that you don't feel great—go out for a walk. Don't miss your exercise—the oxygen and endorphins will help so, so much. And eat like a pregnant woman overcoming morning sickness—small meals 5 times a day—don't let your stomach get empty—helps counter the nausea. Sleep with a banana by the side of your bed and a pitcher of water—hydrate all night long and have the banana in case you are feeling a little queasy first thing in the morning. Demand that your doctor is giving you a wonder drug called Emend—best anti-nausea drug on the market. Insist on it. Look into getting Chia seeds from your health food store or on line. They are flax on steroids. They are wonderful on your oatmeal in the morning and have all the Omega 3s you need and fiber and calcium.

11) Ginger—best natural anti-nausea food. Chop fresh ginger into everything. Eat it raw. Make tea from it. It got so desperate the other day I went straight from the gym to a nearby sushi restaurant to eat a mound of pickled ginger because it was the only thing I could think of to settle my stomach.

Be strong, kick ass and remember this pithy Australian cancer awareness slogan: "Cancer...a word—not a sentence."

Call me if you would like to chat.

You will get through this. Don't let the name Triple Negative scare you. This is beatable.

Love, Jennifer

ATHENA JONES

[My doctor] said, very matter-of-factly, that it was her practice to give women a baseline mammogram at age thirty-five. I truly believe she saved my life.

■ ■ ■

Athena Jones is a CNN national correspondent based in New York. She joined CNN in 2011 as a general assignment reporter, reporting on a wide variety of stories, from breaking news to politics. She previously served as a White House producer for NBC News and began her career reporting in Argentina and Chile.

Some of the women in this book—especially the breast cancer survivors who were diagnosed very young—have had bad experiences with doctors who didn't take them seriously. Athena, who had two breast cancer diagnoses, is not one of them. She credits her forward-thinking gynecologist with saving her life not just once, but twice.

THE DIAGNOSIS
Athena was just thirty-six years old when she received her breast cancer diagnosis.

In September 2012, I had just started dating someone I really liked. I went to see my doctor to get on a new type of birth control, and she had said, very matter-of-factly, that it was her practice to give women a baseline mammogram at age thirty-five. I truly believe she saved my life. I found the second breast cancer, but the first wouldn't even have been found for who knows how long? What thirty-six-year-old is thinking about this?

The first time, it was extensive ductal carcinoma in situ. It was in several places in the left breast, but it wasn't invasive. The X-ray looked like someone had taken a house key and scraped my tissue a little bit. It wasn't like lumps or bumps or pebbles. She explained that rapidly dividing and dying cells are leaving behind these calcified spots. It's remarkable.

That same day, I also got a biopsy. I remember because it was an unpleasant experience. I had to be face down on the table. It seemed like there was a very big needle, and there was a lot of blood. I remember, later on, bleeding through my bandage all over my boyfriend's bed. It wasn't a small puncture.

A few days later, she received the diagnosis while working on a story in Baltimore.

I remember being in a classroom, maybe between shoots. We were waiting for students or something, and the doctor called and told me.

I was shocked. I didn't say anything to my producer. I didn't know how to digest it. At the time I was completely focused on my mother [who lived in Houston, Texas], because around the same time, I had learned she was not going to recover from a rare cancer she had.

I didn't want my mother to try to come and take care of me because that's what she would have done. She really needed her own nurse at that point. My stepfather did medical stuff in Vietnam, helping with surgeries, so he was able to take care of her in a way that other people would have needed a home health care person to do it. So bottom line, I couldn't tell people if I didn't want to tell my mother.

Also, I didn't want to waste my positive energy. There was a part of me that didn't want to have to worry about soothing everyone else who would be overly concerned about me. I thought that that would be an extra burden.

Athena did, however, have to figure out how to tell her still-relatively-new boyfriend.

He had already seen me bleed on his bed, and he understood that something was going on. I remember telling him, I asked him, "Remember that biopsy?" I told him it was noninvasive. Granted, I'm no longer with him, but he was very supportive. He said, "There's no question I'm sticking by you."

THE BATTLE

She was also surrounded by a strong group of friends, many of whom were also journalists.

> I met two plastic surgeons and two breast surgeons. And I had friends come with me to each of those, which is really helpful.
>
> In 2012, one of my friends took notes during meetings. I think we even recorded the doctor. We asked if it was OK. It was really helpful to have [my friend] there because I felt like I had someone else taking back up notes to remember details.

Athena ended up having a double mastectomy with reconstructive surgery. If she had wanted to preserve her healthy breast, she could have tried chemotherapy first, but she was more interested in simply nipping the cancer in the bud—in part because she didn't want to be on serious medications were she to get pregnant in the near future.

> I liked the idea of being able to just wipe the slate clean and not have any of these issues. Also [my breasts] could be more equal. I didn't have very large breasts, and I didn't necessarily want to be like weirdly lopsided.
>
> My ex-boyfriend also put me in touch with a girl he knew who had breast cancer and had gotten it younger than me, so I talked to her on the phone. I also talked to [NBC News correspondent and breast cancer survivor] Andrea Mitchell. She has been super helpful throughout; she even came to the hospital for my first surgery in 2012. I also had her doctor in New York. I don't remember my mastectomy being a heavy, weighty thing.
>
> I had it in December and had the whole month off. It was very easy to hide in that way. And yes, I remember people asking, "Where's Athena?" But mostly no one really knew. I told my mother that same month, when I came home for Christmas. I told her because I wasn't trying to keep it from her; I was trying to keep her from coming to DC for her own good. She died in March of 2013.
>
> I didn't do radiation after consulting about it because my doctor and I felt that after the double mastectomy, I already had a low likelihood for a recurrence, and the radiation would only bring me down a few small

percentage points more. So I decided not to do radiation, which obviously in retrospect might have kept [the cancer] at bay.

In 2015, I felt, in the area of the same boob, what felt like a pea. Maybe a couple of peas. At this point, I was covering the Republicans on the campaign trail. It wasn't a long time before I said, "OK, well, surely this can be anything, but I'm gonna go check it out." So I went to my breast surgeon first, and she was hopeful that it wouldn't be anything. But it was. And this time, it was the invasive kind, which means serious trouble—or serious potential for trouble. There must've been a few cells left behind [after the double mastectomy] that continued to grow based on the hormones throughout my body.

Doctors were sad for me. And they were as surprised as I was. You might find it odd, but I wasn't scared for my life. I was really annoyed. I know that sounds like I'm diminishing it, but that's how I felt. I was like, "This again? Are you kidding me?" Having full knowledge of the chemo I was going have to go through, I wasn't thinking, "Oh no, I'm going to die." I was thinking, "This is incredibly disruptive. I'm annoyed."

Athena was thirty-nine years old. Recurrence after a double mastectomy is not common, but it does sometimes happen.[19] This time, she had invasive, triple-positive cancer in the same breast where the DCIS had been. First, Athena had surgery to remove the cancer and her first implant (she later had a second reconstruction). Then, for four and a half months, she had chemotherapy every three weeks, always on a Friday.

I talked to [CNN president] Jeff Zucker, who had had [colon] cancer also twice in his thirties. He told me that he always had his chemo on Fridays, which I was already planning to do. That way I could recover all weekend; I had time to rest. The first four of them, I brought a friend. They took off the afternoon and they came with me. One of them introduced me to *Fixer Upper* on HGTV.

Athena fared well with chemotherapy, except for a few physical changes.

The biggest problem for me with chemo was that I thought I gained weight from steroids, and I couldn't do yoga because I was wearing a braided wig. I did Flywheel instead of yoga because I couldn't turn upside down at Flywheel [and risk the wig falling off]. I also probably did Flywheel at times [in the middle of the day] when no one would ever be there [so she wouldn't risk running into someone she knew—Washington is a very small town that way].

During radiation, I had an issue with lymphedema. My arm didn't blow up to the size of my thigh or anything, but my rings wouldn't fit and my hands would get tight. It ended up going away.

But the most visceral part of Athena's chemo experience was the loss of her hair.

I wore a braided wig, which the most part worked fine. But some viewers noticed. I remember being in a wig in Japan on an Obama trip to Hiroshima, and I remember some person on the Internet saying, "That's horrible, what does she have on her head?" So there were definitely people who noticed. But my colleagues were mostly not black people. Most of the people who I came across were not people who were going to notice that it was a braided wig. Thank God.

These days when people make comments about certain things, I will gently explain to them why things are the way they are. Some people have commented on my Facebook page about how I should be a better example to young black girls, that their hair as it grows naturally is good enough, and I have to explain to them, "I know where you're coming from, but this is the option for me because I'm a two-time cancer survivor." But at the time [during chemo], I didn't want to reveal myself to defend myself—especially to someone I didn't even know.

My goal was that, after chemo, my hair would grow enough that I could put my braids back in. I was looking forward to all these natural hairstyles that I was going to rock. Then I put the braids back in, and the front of my hair, which is where I have these continued problems, was too delicate. The first set of braids I did after my hair grew back enough, that hair never really recovered.

I've been doing a million things to try to get my hair to grow. And that's why I wear a weave now. The second time I went back for braids, my hairdresser was like, "I don't want to do it. I can't. We shouldn't do this because it's not going to work." She was the one who coaxed me into getting a weave. I just wish I had had some knowledge going into it. But you don't know what you don't know. So I didn't know to ask.

■

I wasn't thinking, "Oh no, I'm going to die." I was

thinking, "This is incredibly disruptive. I'm annoyed."

■

THE COMEBACK

Professionally, Athena was disappointed to lose her chance at covering the campaign. But her new beat, the White House early shift, worked out incredibly well.

I was really excited to be on the campaign trail. I was mostly covering Republicans. I did a lot of Jeb Bush and Marco Rubio events. I did Trump events. This was all in the primaries, of course.

As importantly, I was covering the debates. I was usually the *New Day* person [reporting on the debates for the CNN morning show]. I had hoped and planned that this was all going to continue and that I would be active on the campaign trail throughout the election, but that is not what happened. I had to leave the campaign trail, but work was incredibly accommodating by posting me at the White House on a permanent early shift, so that I could be in town to go to chemo every three weeks. I was always out of work by like 1:00 p.m. at the latest. [That routine continued with her radiation treatments once chemo was done.]

I like to always try to look on the bright side, though. I was happy that, number one, I would have a somewhat predictable schedule. But also, I knew plenty of sources at the White House, so I was already in a good position that way. And I was there in the very beginning of the Obama

2008 campaign, so for me, it was really nice being able to come back around. And I remember one day covering an event in the Roosevelt Room [of the White House]. President Obama saw me, that I was back, and acknowledged me. It was cool.

I think, in the end, I was really very satisfied. I mean, it's a pretty cool beat. It was almost like a blessing in disguise. There were a lot of hard things about it, but I was able to come full circle. And it was great.

I've been cancer free since 2016 and I'm still dealing with the aftereffects [of hair loss] and going to great lengths. That part is annoying. I do have a very good solution now, but I'm still not fully back to my old self. I am a new self.

JOAN LUNDEN

I always like to tell women who are newly diagnosed or
going through breast cancer treatment that it's hard to
see the light at the end of the tunnel. But look at me.
I'm the light at the end of the tunnel.

■ ■ ■

Joan Lunden is an award-winning journalist, motivational speaker, and
women's health advocate who spent nearly two decades as a host on
ABC's *Good Morning America*. She is the author of twelve books and is
now a special correspondent on the *TODAY Show*. She is also the mother
of seven children, including two sets of twins.

Joan has conducted thousands of interviews with all sorts of people
on a wide variety of topics. It's a perk of the job, talking to people who
are passionate about issues you often don't know anything about. But at
the same time, it means that sometimes you can't relate to the story or
interview on certain levels because they're so far removed from your
own personal experience and background. It doesn't make them better
or worse; it just makes them different.

But the interview Joan did in 2009 with renowned breast cancer expert Dr. Susan Love, on a show she was doing called *Health Corner*, was—
quite literally—news she could use, even if she didn't realize it at the
time. And she thinks some of what she learned during that interview
helped to catch her breast cancer earlier than she would have.

THE DIAGNOSIS

Joan didn't have a family history of cancer, so she wasn't particularly
concerned about her breast health when she talked to Dr. Love.

The interview was about mammograms, but since I didn't have any breast cancer in my family history, I felt like it wasn't going to be my problem. As I finished the interview with Dr. Love, she asked if I got mammograms regularly. I told her that I found them stressful because I was always called back in for more pictures. And when that happens, your first reaction is, "Do you see something bad?" They'd always tell me, "Don't worry, it's just that we can't see anything because you have very dense breasts."

Dr. Love told me that I should also be getting an ultrasound, because dense tissue shows up white on a mammogram, and so does cancer, and that makes it difficult to see cancer. I was shocked. No doctor of mine had ever told me that before.

As a journalist, sometimes we do stories that impact us in such a way that when we come back home, we act on them personally. Thankfully, this time I did. If I hadn't been sent to do that interview, I wouldn't have known to ask for that ultrasound.

The ultrasound she had in 2014 caught two separate tumors which, after a core biopsy, were confirmed to be cancerous. While one tumor was DCIS and thus considered early stage, the diagnosis for the second tumor was triple-negative, meaning her breast cancer would not respond to the targeted therapies used to confront the three common triggers of the cancer cells' growth.

When I first heard that I was "triple negative," I thought that sounded good—at least I was negative to three things. Then the doctor explained that it meant I didn't have any of the receptors for targeted therapy and would need months of chemotherapy followed by radiation and surgery. Since then, there's been incredible advances and they are developing targeted therapy for triple-negative breast cancer, but they didn't have it in 2014.

When you are diagnosed with breast cancer, it feels like you've been shot out of a cannon with information coming at you at supersonic speed. My diagnosis was shocking to me because of the lack of family history, but I've since learned that fewer than 15 percent of women diagnosed with breast cancer have a family history.[20] Had I known that, I wouldn't have been so nonchalant.

Joan was familiar with breaking all sorts of news to a television audience. But she was unsure of how to handle this very personal, very difficult, report.

> When I received my diagnosis, I really didn't want to tell anyone. Picking up the phone and saying to friends, "I have cancer" was incredibly difficult. Maybe it's my age, but I come from an era when women never told anyone they had breast cancer, and it certainly wasn't something that you spoke about publicly. I know people who have had breast cancer and didn't tell their children. That's what it used to be like. There was a time when cancer was spoken of in hush hush terms as the "Big C."

Joan thought about her father, Dr. Erle Blunden (ABC removed the "B" from Joan's last name), who was tragically killed in a plane crash when Lunden was thirteen.

> I was so young when my father passed away that I wanted to know more about him and his life. So a few years ago, I spoke with some of my father's colleagues about his career and what medicine and cancer treatment was like back in that time. I learned that sometimes they didn't even tell women that they had cancer. They explained that they didn't have all the treatments that are available today, that there was only surgery. If the cancer was found in a late stage and nothing could be done to save their lives, it was thought that telling them would only upset them. I was flabbergasted.
>
> Betty Ford was the first woman to come out publicly and talk about having breast cancer and made it OK for other women to talk about breast cancer. I do think that today, there's still that little hangover of feeling like you shouldn't say anything, at least that's what I felt in those first moments. Not to mention, I'd written six books on health! So I also worried that I'd let people down. I thought, "Did I bring this on?"
>
> I remember walking out of the radiology lab after my ultrasound, it was hard to even dial my husband from the car and say those words, "I have breast cancer."
>
> Yes, I'm a bit of a Type A personality. Sometimes I might think of myself as Superwoman, so I had a difficult time feeling as if I was in the victim

role. I even felt like I was, in a way, letting my husband down. I'd always thought of myself as this incredibly healthy, strong woman. My husband is younger than me—ten years younger—but I've always felt like it didn't make any difference because I'm a mover, a doer, and a healthy person. Now all of a sudden, I wasn't.

Nobody could ask for a more supportive husband than I have. He jumped in and said "This doesn't define you, you're going to fight this, you're going to beat this, and life will go on." It's hard to imagine that when you're right at that stage.

She thought about the good she could do if she brought along her fans and viewers, the people who had been tuning into her for their news for all these years, for her breast cancer journey.

It took about 24 hours, maybe 48 hours, for me to wake up to the fact that I had lived my entire life in the public eye. I shared everything. They watched me go through every pregnancy—everything! And whether I liked it or not, every nuance of my life was consumed and often critiqued by the public. However, here was a chapter of my life that if I shared it, could perhaps help others battling cancer.

I had always thought I was going to be a doctor like my dad but had never fulfilled that dream. I took psychology in college because being a psych major was the closest I felt I could get to being a doctor—which, by the way, likely helped me in my interviews over the years—but I'd always had that inner desire to follow in his footsteps. For years I had reveled in doing all the health segments on *GMA*. When I left *GMA*, all of the projects I chose were health oriented. I even started my website called Joan Lunden's Healthy Living. So, I thought, "It might seem a little odd, but the universe just dropped an opportunity in my lap to go out and disseminate health information and maybe even save a life. Isn't that pretty much following in your dad's footsteps? Isn't that carrying on his legacy?" Of course it was, and it was something that really did change my life.

She thought hard about how she wanted to reveal her news to the world. She began talking to friend and current *GMA* host Robin Roberts, who had joined the show in 2005 and shared her battle with breast cancer. Robin also ended up having a rare bone marrow disease that she shared with her television audience. It became clear to Joan that the obvious place to make her announcement would be alongside Robin and co-host Amy Robach, also a breast cancer survivor.

I called Robin and Robin said, "You need to get this two-thousand-pound elephant off your shoulders. As soon as you say the words out loud, you won't feel the pressure. It won't be easy, but I'll be there with you. You've got to do this before someone sees you at a cancer center and then the tabloid headline might be 'JOAN LUNDEN IS DYING OF CANCER.' Beat them to the punch."

Two days later I was scheduled on the program. I told Robin that I didn't want to come in to the studio early because I knew everybody was going to say, "How are you? What are you talking about today?" Robin assured me that the only other person that would know why I was there would be the producer.

The producers and crew in the room gave her an ovation at the end of the interview.

It was a relief to be honest with everyone, but it was also scary as hell. Because, again, I felt like I was letting people down. I was also sharing with the world—and I'd shared everything with them—but still, I was sharing with the world that I had this compromised health. I had to say those words. "I have cancer." And it was really hard. But Robin was right. As soon as I did it, it was like I had my freedom to walk out of there and take a deep breath and exhale and move forward and do what I needed to do.

THE BATTLE

Joan quickly got to work finding the physicians that she wanted in charge of her care. She got several opinions, and they diverged. One oncologist recommended a traditional approach of surgery first, followed by chemo. However, another oncologist advocated for a neoadjuvant approach, beginning with chemotherapy to shrink the tumor and then moving on to surgery. They would also be adding a drug called carboplatin, which studies had shown to be effective against triple-negative breast cancer.

I don't know if it's because I am from an earlier generation or if it's because my dad was a cancer surgeon, but in my day, nobody ever questioned a doctor. But my daughter Lindsay said, "In today's world you always go for [a] second opinion, and we are going." But of course, what you get is just that: a second, and often different opinion. This can be confusing for patients, because it's then up to you to choose how to proceed with your cancer treatment. Picking the right strategy is very scary. You think, "What if I make the wrong decision?"

Joan chose the neoadjuvant approach. The chemotherapy shrunk her tumor by 95 percent. It meant that she ended up having a small lumpectomy, to remove the triple-negative tumor and the DCIS, rather than a more invasive operation, which would have likely required a lot of reconstructive surgeries.

As it happened, my cancer was practically gone by the time I had my surgery. Is one breast slightly smaller than the other? Sure. Does it bother me enough to do anything about it? No.

Ever the reporter, Joan brought her iPhone into every medical setting she was allowed to, documenting the entire process, including talking about her fears about chemo—she wasn't a fan of the needles or the prospect of hair loss—and before and after her procedure to get a port installed, which allowed her chemotherapy to be administered in a more major vein than those in her arm.

Is one breast slightly smaller than the other? Sure.

Does it bother me enough to do anything about it? No.

Joan also started doing more TV interviews, realizing the power she had in her platform. Most of the time, she received positive feedback. But it was also through those TV appearances that she developed a deeper understanding of the privilege she possessed going into her diagnosis, not just in terms of being a financially secure woman with access to good health care, but also someone with a loving family and extensive support system.

One day, close to the end of my chemo, I was on *Access Hollywood*, and they had questions that had been submitted from their audience. One of the questions was, "What do you think has helped you get through your cancer battle?" And my answer, on-air, was that my family and friends being there for me had really gotten me through the tough times. Even though I always protested and told them I can do this myself, they would always come with me and, truth be told, in the end I was really happy that they were there.

That evening I was reading my Facebook messages, and this one woman wrote to me and said, "I saw you on *Access Hollywood* today and I just want you to be mindful of the fact that there are a lot of us out here who are working hard to get all of our chemo appointments in while still cooking dinner for our kids at night and working to keep a roof over our heads, and we don't have that same kind of support system that you're talking about, and when I hear you say that [about your friends and family], it made me cry. So, I'm so happy that you're doing well and that you have had that family around you, but I think it's important, because you're on the air all the time, that you keep in mind that there are a lot of us out here that don't have that, and it makes us feel sad when you say that."

After taking five minutes to dry my tears, I realized I was so glad she sent it to me because she really gave me a dose of reality for many people. She made me incredibly mindful of how difficult this is for so many women across the country. And I'm not only speaking about the single, working mom like this woman was. It can be any woman who is trying to navigate life. Any mom at home with kids, or woman trying to maintain a relationship, or keep a job. Because my experience has been so public, my experience has become not just my own, but a compilation of so many women out there. Every single day that I share this journey with others and I hear back from all of them, I feel that we are all in it together somehow. That woman really gave me a huge reminder, as I'm out talking about it all the time, to remember that there's a lot of women out there like her.

THE COMEBACK

Hearing from women across the country made Joan very cognizant that many women don't have the resources that she had, even with intangible things like familial love. That's why she has tried to take advantage of every opportunity to get her message out there, and to use those resources for good.

Every single day that I share this journey with others

and I hear back from all of them, I feel that we are all

in it together somehow.

One of the most powerful examples of that was her September 2014 appearance, bald, on the cover of *People Magazine* that really propelled a conversation about breast health and breast density into the public's consciousness.

It's a striking picture—one you might actually remember seeing when the issue was first published. Joan is in a white button-down shirt, with the collar cheekily popped. She's wearing diamond rings on both her fingers, diamond earrings, and a fresh manicure. Her makeup is simple but glowing. Her smile is radiant. And her head is bare. The caption reads, "I WILL BEAT THIS."

I've had a wonderful relationship with *People Magazine* over the years, and with editor Kate Coyne. But when she called and said they wanted to do a cover, at first I was reluctant. But Kate said, "We'll do the photographs with a wig on, we'll do it with a nice scarf, and then if you're up to it that day, we'll do it just bald. Then I will let you make the decision as to what to do. I'll be there with you. I think this can be an amazingly impactful story."

Now, at that point in time, I didn't even know that I had this unbelievable message to deliver about the importance of understanding your breast density. That came to me as I accrued more knowledge over the coming months, thankfully, in time for the interview I did with her.

After discussing it with my family, and thinking long and hard about the decision, the day of the shoot arrived, and I still was unsure of what I was going to do. The team at *People* had chosen [acclaimed photographer] Ruven Afanador to do this cover, but I was a little concerned about how I would feel taking my wig off in front of him. But he was terrific. When the time came for me to take the wig off, I asked for everyone to clear the room. My daughter Sarah, who was there, said, "I'm going to stay in the room. I just want to be there for you."

I took the wig off, and he brought the camera in so close that it was intimidating. I felt totally exposed. But I just thought to myself, "If you've ever dug down deep and pulled a smile out of your heart, this is the time you've got to do that." Since then, I've had women say to me, "I just got diagnosed. And as I heard those words from the doctor, 'you have cancer,' I thought about your *People Magazine* picture. But it wasn't your bald head; it was the smile on your face that said to me, 'I can beat this. I can get through this.'"

When I hear those sentiments from people, I feel it was definitely worth it. I had been concerned because I didn't want people to think I was being opportunistic. But nobody did. It was totally taken in the proper way. In fact, there was an amazing heartening reaction to it, and it was a jumping off point for where my career would go next and much of my advocacy work. I've probably given a hundred speeches in the last four years to breast cancer organizations. As I've traveled the country to speak, I've often asked audiences, "How many women in this room know their breast density?" There have been times when no one raised their hand. That's when I've realized that I need to be out there. I need to be talking about this. And frankly, I think that it helped me in my own personal journey because I wasn't just wallowing in my own diagnosis and my own treatment. I had changed my focus from my own breast cancer to *the* fight against breast cancer, and it made my cancer journey so much more meaningful.

I always like to tell women who are newly diagnosed or going through it, "It's hard to see the light at the end of the tunnel. But look at me. I'm the light at the end of the tunnel. Here I am. It wasn't the easiest road, but other women have it much worse than I have. I got through it and I hardly think about it anymore."

Everyone will tell you that you go into cancer one person and you come out another, and I am here to tell you that it's true. You come out appreciating life in a different way; you come out cognizant of your health and how important it is to protect it; you come out truly understanding what family and friends will do for you, how they will come to your aid. It's important that we allow those who love us, to have a chance to love and care for us. It is an opportunity that not everybody gets.

GERRI WILLIS

I thought medical stuff was way over my head, and I
wouldn't be a part of it. I thought, "You just do it to me,
and I'll be back later." But that's not the way this works.
You have to be part of it.

■ ■ ■

Gerri Willis joined FOX Business Network in 2010 and is an anchor and
personal finance reporter. Before joining FBN, she served as the personal finance editor for CNN Business News and hosted the weekly half-
hour show *Your Bottom Line*. She is the author of four books, including
Rich Is Not a Four-Letter Word.

THE DIAGNOSIS

In 2016, Gerri was just about to begin promoting her newly published
book when she started feeling something strange in her breast. It was a
hardness, flat and oblong. It wasn't a cherry or pea-shaped lump, as she
had been advised to look out for, but it hadn't been there before. She
knew she had to get it checked out, but she decided she would wait until the book was released and she had done a week's worth of promotion.
Then her nipple inverted.

Here's the really bad part about this and what I want people to hear: I
had my first mammogram six months before diagnosis. I had never had
one. You have to get mammograms! You have to be tested. But that mammogram came up clear. So then I went back to get my nipple checked out.
I was still living in a dream world when my doctor said, "You need to go
have this tested." I said, "Next Tuesday looks good," and she said, "No,
right now."

Gerri went to another location for a sonogram and, ultimately, a biopsy.

> When I saw the nurses and their reaction to me when they were ana-lyzing the sonogram, there was none of the upbeat chatter of, "Well, you know, this looks OK." It was very silent and quiet, so I knew something was going on.
>
> The next week, after they had run all these tests, I got a call from my primary care physician, and she said, "Gerri, your tests came back positive." I said, "Do you mean I have breast cancer?" And she said, "Yes, you do." I was deflated, but I still was not taking all this in. It took a very long time for me to think that something could go physically wrong with my body because I just never had had anything—I mean, flu, colds. I had never broken a bone. It was very difficult for me to in-ternalize and accept.

Gerri was diagnosed with stage III lobular carcinoma, which, she learned, is harder to detect on a mammogram. As one medical study put it, tumors in the breast ducts tend to form glandular structures, while lobular tumors "are less cohesive and tend to invade in single file."[21] But for Gerri, what she calls her "turning point"—the moment she realized just what she was facing—didn't take place until a while after her diagnosis.

> I first went to the woman who would do the mastectomy on me, a fabulous surgeon at Memorial Sloan Kettering. You know when you meet somebody who's at the top of their game and just on it? She was that person. But I told her, "I want to get rid of it." I was just thinking, "How do we get through this as fast as we can?" And I spoke with [FOX Pen-tagon correspondent and survivor] Jennifer Griffin. She told me, "The thing you don't know, that nobody tells you, that you've really got to prepare yourself for, is that it takes a long time. You get through the mastectomy, and then you're onto chemo. And then you're onto breast reconstruction. And then you're on to radiation. It's really a long process. It takes forever. Everything you do has implications for your body, and you have reactions to it."

THE BATTLE

Gerri had a mastectomy followed by chemotherapy, then reconstructive surgery between chemo and radiation.

The first two chemo treatments, which was the Red Devil—the really heavy stuff [Adriamycin]—I kind of sailed through that. And I thought, "This is not so bad." Third chemo—oh my God! It was like getting hit by a baseball bat. And that really was my turning point to get my head together on this. I go in for the very last Red Devil treatment, and it just really messes with your veins. They collapse. And I didn't have a port. So they're poking, over and over again, trying to find a vein, and I hate needles. They were bringing nurses in from other floors, asking, "Can you try? Can you try?" I was just so tense. My shoulders are at my ears, my whole body is tense and nervous and anxious. And just seeing that red stuff go into your [veins] is creepy.

And then finally I thought, "These women are not here to kill you. They're here to administer a drug that you need to survive. You better co-operate with them. This could be your best day of treatment or it could be your worst—it's up to you. You make the choice! You're driving the car! Come on now!" So I relaxed, and that needle went in on the next try.

From that point on, instead of thinking about the whole arc of treatment, I started thinking step-by-step-by-step. I got a big whiteboard for my office at home, and I wrote, in every threshold, every step I was going to take. I listed all the chemos I had lined up and everything after that, and I would check everything off. Everything was color-coded. The steps would be in blue and the checkmarks would be in red.

This was a complete remake of the way I thought about myself and what I was doing and how to move forward. Because this required that I break [each goal] into very small steps so that I could emotionally handle what was going on. We're going to this chemotherapy session, and then we're making dinner. And it became very simple. Every time I hit one of those milestones, one of those goals—even if it was a very small step—I'd pat myself on the back.

So you're moving forward, getting involved with every step, living in the moment. And that's the most critical thing: enjoying where you are and what you're doing and taking it all in.

By the time I hit radiation, which is a daily thing, the whiteboard is full, and I'm marking [treatments] off one by one. Instead of just being oriented to those daily goals, now I'm getting to know everybody on the radiation team. Now it's about relationships, so I looked forward to going. It was the highlight of my day, getting over there. I got to know the technicians. We decorated the radiation machine for Christmas. I went over with presents. I was living that moment. I mean, you have to be part of the treatment. You have to be your own doctor in some ways. You have to know what's going on with your body, and you have to be alert and in the game.

I thought medical stuff was way over my head, and I wouldn't be a part of it. But that's not the way this works. You have to be part of it.

Part of that commitment to being fully in the game meant that Gerri had to cut back on work. That was one of the biggest challenges for her, because up until that point, work was life. Executive Bill Shine, who later left the network over his handling of sexual harassment allegations there, was extremely supportive, calling Gerri every month to check in and encouraging her to take as much time as she needed before she returned to work.

People in the office were amazing. [FOX host] Neil Cavuto was very, very supportive. Management was supportive. That's their MO there. That's one thing that they are known for. If you have some major problem, and you're part of the FOX family, they are very supportive. One of the managers in FOX Business had had a cancer death very close to him, and he was constantly watching out for me. "Do you really need to come back? I don't think you really need to come back," he would say. "It's all going to be here when you come back."

I couldn't imagine being out of work for a long time. I was the kind of person who didn't really take a lot of vacation time, and I was there every day, so it was unimaginable to me that I could be gone for months on end. And the big mistake I made, frankly, is I kept saying I was going to be back and couldn't make it back.

I kept saying, "Well, I'll be back after the mastectomy and then I'll go out for chemo." And then, during chemo it was like, "I'll be back right after chemo." Actually, no, you're not going to be right back after chemo. I kept making that error over and over again, misunderstanding how long it would take my body to heal.

I was very optimistic about how long it would take me to get back. Part of it was just blind stupidity, frankly. I had never been through anything like this before. I had not seen it up close in my family. You hear about people who like run marathons when they're in chemo. I was not that person.

[At work,] you're out there all the time, you're talking to people all the time, you're in the mix, interviewing people, thinking about stories, and then you get pulled away from that for this, and suddenly, I was on my own in a way that I never am typically in a business day. And I had a lot of time to think.

She also had to deal with losing her hair.

For better or worse, my hair was part of my performance, part of my image. It could have been grace, it could have been wit, but it was my hair, unfortunately. I was directed to a wigmaker in Stanford, Connecticut, and she said, "Don't buzz your head." She advised against it, which I regretted because then you're walking around the house pulling your own hair out.

[There's] this special process by which they save your hair by freezing your scalp while you're sitting in chemo. It's this wild new thing. It's expensive. And I considered it, but then I realized, "OK, what's important here? It's getting through the treatment. Who cares about the hair?"

On the plus side, being out of the office allowed Gerri to spend more time with her loved ones, including her husband, David, and her brother, Steve.

David understood at a very gut level that your self-confidence is very important to whatever's going on. So it was always just base-level support—no shock, no anger, no fear coming from him, ever.

My brother, who is a Presbyterian minister, deals with people in this situation all the time, and he's used to it. [But] he comes up to visit our place up in the Berkshires, and there's that moment—I'm past mid-chemo, I've lost twenty pounds—and I could tell from his face: He could barely look at me because I was so changed in the way I looked. But we had the most astonishing time together, and we weren't talking about old times. It was more about getting to know the adult of the person I grew up with.

He gave me great advice on how to calm my fears, and relax, and open up to the world. He was this wonderful spiritual guide, my brother the minister. And we spent like three days together, I think just the two of us.

He and I did a lot of walking together. It was just very relaxing and very nurturing. Being in nature is a huge thing. My memories of the strongest emotions I had during treatment were gratitude, just being awe-struck by the beauty of things, feeling overwhelmed by how many wonderful things there are in the world.

THE COMEBACK

When Gerri was ready to return to work, she had gone through a profound personal transformation.

I went through a very long period of just gratitude, and general happiness, and feeling upbeat. Every day's a gift, dammit! You may not have tomorrow. And finding that out firsthand is really a gift.

She'd gone through some physical changes too. For starters, her chest had grown. She had only removed one breast, but ended up having to get plastic surgery on both.

The first time I go to see the cosmetic surgeon who's going to redo my breast, first his nurse walks in with this big book with pictures of women from their neck to their waist. And I'm looking at that and thinking, "Not one of those will fit on my torso!" So he comes in, examines me, and says, "Well, Gerri, what I have to tell you is that we really can't reconstruct breasts as small as yours." I'm like, "Everybody's a complainer." Then he said, "We have to make them bigger." So I had both sides done.

She also began sporting a new pixie cut.

[When I returned to the air] I went and got a wig. And the pictures of me in that wig store are like [sad trombone]. I was wearing it for a long time and it looked OK, and then suddenly I felt like I had a possum on my head, and I hated it. I began to hate this wig more than anything in the world. Our hair and makeup people, who were unbelievable through all of this, were like, "You have to get rid of this because you look better without it." And I never would have done it without their encouragement.

We did this unveiling [of my new pixie cut] on Kennedy's show. It allowed me to talk about the process and try to convince people to get the mammogram and not be afraid of the treatment, because for me it was actually a year of stupendous growth and personal fulfillment. But the whole hair story is hysterical, because it was so stupid that it was such a big thing.

I feel like I'm more myself now with this than I was with the long, heavy, big hair. I feel like this is more me.

■

Every day's a gift, dammit! You may not have

tomorrow. And finding that out firsthand is really a gift.

■

Most importantly, Gerri's breast cancer journey enhanced her personal relationships—particularly her relationship with her husband.

I mean, frankly, in many ways, this experience was a gift for me and really brought me closer to family, closer to my husband. We've always had a great relationship but this was like, we're now at a level we'd never been at before. And it's because of this!

Although Gerri's breast cancer is still in remission, she remains vigilant about her health. In January 2020, she announced that she was taking a leave of absence to have a prophylactic hysterectomy after a routine PAP smear revealed pre-cancerous cells on her cervix. Gerri used her visibility in the media to educate parents and women about the importance of routine screenings and the HPV vaccine Gardasil. On FoxNews.com, she writes:

Early detection is critical. Please, take my advice, ladies. I know it can be hard to find the time for these simple tests but your life may quite literally depend on it.

PART VI

THE
HEALERS

THERE IS A biblical proverb that urges, "physician, heal thyself." In other words, it's important to look inward and address the problems within oneself before trying to help solve the problems of others. The proverb is intended as a moral reminder, but it's also a concept that rings true for the two physicians in this chapter, both breast specialists whose understanding of the disease deepened after they themselves were diagnosed. They were already skilled doctors with expertise in their fields, but getting diagnosed with breast cancer gave them a unique perspective on their specialty that, thankfully, relatively few doctors are privy to.

Other women have dedicated their lives to healing in a broader sense. Breast cancer survivors Sally Oren and Ellen Noghès began an informal diplomatic breast cancer club to provide emotional healing within the Washington, D.C., ambassadorial community. And Geeta Rao Gupta drew strength from her team of employees focused on international aid in order to confront her own illness.

Though they have taken different paths, the women in this chapter have all devoted themselves to healing the wounds of women around the world—both physical and otherwise. And they do it so well because they have had to patch up their wounds themselves.

DR. KIMBERLY ALLISON

If you have a good network of people around you, they want to help you in some way and not just be crying on the phone. And it's nice to let them. For them and you.

■ ■ ■

Dr. Kimberly Allison, director of breast pathology at Stanford, only learned of the discipline of pathology about halfway through medical school. You could call it "love at first slide." In layman's terms, pathology is the practice of examining body tissue for diagnosis. That definition might sound a bit dry, but for Kimberly, looking at each piece of breast tissue under a microscope was like putting together a puzzle, where you don't know what the finished product is going to look like until you fit every piece together.

She was in charge of recognizing patterns in cells which could then help a patient's doctors figure out what sort of treatment that patient was likely to respond well to. She'd present her findings at what's known as tumor board, where physicians and specialists from all sorts of disciplines gather together to discuss the best course of action for an individual patient, based on all the disparate pieces of information they'd collected. The pathology reports were always some of the longest, but they were also among the most impactful.

Breast cancer is a more complicated puzzle to solve every time. There's not as many diagnoses but you were a really big part of the treatment team. At tumor board, all of the little details in our pathology reports make big treatment differences.

But then, to be honest, there was also more of a clinical need for me in breast [pathology], so that ended up being what I focused in. It wasn't because of a family history or some backstory or my own diagnosis, because I hadn't had it yet.

That all changed once it was Kimberly's own tissue under the microscope.

THE DIAGNOSIS

Like FOX Pentagon correspondent Jennifer Griffin (see page 171), Kimberly discovered something abnormal in her breast while nursing her second child.

> I noticed there was a firm area. It wasn't even really a lump; it was a shelf-like area in the upper aspect of my left breast. And I really didn't think much of it. When you're breastfeeding, your breasts go through changes. They can be totally lumpy and bumpy, and there's all sorts of funny things that you don't want to freak out about. But I did go into my OB-GYN and say, "Hey what do you think of this?" Luckily, she didn't send me away. She said, "Yeah, this is a little funny, I don't like it. Let's get a mammogram." She got me a mammogram, but when you're breastfeeding, it's completely white, so there really wasn't much to see, so they did an ultrasound and said, "OK, there's a big mass. It could be nothing, it could be breastfeeding-related changes, or it could be something worse." And they asked, "Would you like a biopsy or not?" I said, "Yes, I'd love to see my own cells under a microscope, that would be cool!"
>
> Then the next day [my colleague] definitely took a little bit of time, and I got to feel that angst of, "I'm waiting for a diagnosis, what's it going to be?"
>
> She came to my door with a colleague, and I saw the two of them together and thought, "Oh God. They're there to help deliver bad news." They told me the diagnosis, and they were very upset. I was shocked because I thought, "This cannot be happening to me. This is what I do for a living. I don't have any family history of this. I'm super healthy." But of course, most breast cancers are random, so it isn't something that you can predict.

She found out that she had stage III, HER2-positive, hormone receptor-negative breast cancer, which means the cancer was bigger than 5 centimeters, had spread to her lymph nodes, and was growing fast.

I learned from the process about what it's like to be on the other side of things: Right after your diagnosis, you're in such a panicked and fragile state, where you're imagining all the possibilities out there. And [once] you get in to see somebody who can even address your fears and come up with a plan, so that you're not in this limbo and you feel some sense of control, you become a lot calmer.

But that fear of the unknown is the worst state to be in—at least it was for me.

Kimberly was more nervous about handling the emotions of her four-year-old daughter. She struggled with figuring out how to tell her and how much she should know. She wanted her to be aware, given all of the physical changes she knew she would experience. So she tried to deliver the news in an upbeat way.

The baby—she had no idea was going on. But I was really worried what my four-year-old would think when I told her, and how could I tell her, and what would she understand. And I didn't want her to get overly emotional because I didn't have enough information, because you don't know if you're going to survive.

I tried to tell it to her in an upbeat way, like, "They found something in Mommy that needs to be fixed, I'm going to need to take medicine that's going to make me sick, make me lose my hair." And she immediately focused in on the hair, and said, "And it'll grow back like grass?" She totally pictured Mom as a Chia Pet.

THE BATTLE

Like all new breast cancer patients, Kimberly had to choose the treatment team who would guide her through the process. In her case, they were all her colleagues.

I knew I wanted to be treated where I was working, because I trusted everybody there so much. Maybe it put them in an awkward position when I said, "I'd like you to be my surgeon, I'd like you to be my oncologist." I didn't really give them the option to say no, and I probably should have, but they were all great. They met with me and my husband and went through what the treatment plan was going to be. I didn't have a lot of different options because it was an aggressive form, and it was pretty clear what I needed. But I felt lucky that I knew my team well rather than having to shop around for a lot of opinions and make sure that I was getting the best care.

She knew that the specifics of her cancer meant she was going to need chemotherapy plus the drug Herceptin, which was shown to be effective against HER2-positive breast cancer, and she opted for neoadjuvant therapy.

That's a big thing to jump right into. And I think I started on April Fools' Day too, which just felt really cruel.

I had three months of Adriamycin and Cytoxan. Adriamycin is the "Red Devil"—or the "Red Sunshine," depending on how you think about it. And that was the one I was most nervous about. It's tougher juice. I was on a regimen where you got a smaller dose every week, so it wasn't so horrible. And I had a lot of side effect medications upfront which made it really pretty manageable. I'd recently been pregnant, and as I was going through chemotherapy in the beginning, I was like, "God, being pregnant I felt a little bit worse!"

I had three months of Adriamycin and Cytoxan and then had Taxol for the next three months plus Herceptin, the antibody therapy. That's given [via] IV too, and then, when you finish your six months of therapy, you continue the Herceptin for another almost a year. You go back every three weeks and get this injection that doesn't take as long, and you can leave thirty minutes later.

Chemotherapy's come a long way. I was really terrified of it, but it really is so much better managed than it used to be. Getting chemotherapy for breast cancer is not getting a bone marrow transplant. You're not being snowed with it until you have no immune cells left. You're basically living your life. I was still going to work three days a week. I went in to get chemotherapy on Wednesdays and I'd take Thursdays off, and the other days I was at work. It was powerful in that way: It slowed you down, and I am a high-speed person who doesn't slow down easily.

I'd recently been pregnant, and as I was going through
chemotherapy in the beginning, I was like, "God,
being pregnant I felt a little bit worse!"

Following her chemotherapy, she took a six-week break, then had her bilateral mastectomy with reconstruction, and then began radiation. For someone like Kimberly, it was different to just step back and let the treatment run its course.

One of the hardest things about cancer is you can't work hard at it and win. There are so many other things in my life I could just work harder at, and I could achieve more. And with cancer you can't just do a good job and survive. A lot of it is luck and giving up control. I really meditated a lot on that: "OK, medicine do your job. This is not in my control." I think there are a lot of little things you can do as a cancer patient to feel like you have some control. You have your treatment plan, and you can believe in it. That's a choice you make. And then you can take care of the rest of yourself. For a little while I gave up sugar, but I got off that bandwagon. I started doing yoga and meditating. I started walking every day. I used to run but I just wanted to be outside every day for a little bit. There's spiritual healing. I saw a shaman, and if you're religious you can go to your religious community. I didn't really have one, so I was experimenting with lots of different spiritual paths. I think that lack of control is really terrifying, and there's lots of different ways you can embrace it without giving up.

It was very important to Kimberly to keep on a steady work schedule, even if she was cutting back.

For me coming to work was almost in a weird way an escape from my own situation, although ironically, I was looking at breast cancer all day.

My director asked me if I wanted to keep specializing in breast pathology. Did I want to switch to, like, prostate, because I can't get that? But it made me realize how passionate I am about my job, that I wanted to keep doing it.

I had the complication of, just two weeks before [the diagnosis], having been appointed the director of breast pathology because my former mentor had left unexpectedly. I was pretty junior when I got that role, and now I was going to be undergoing cancer treatment. They wondered, "Is she going to be able to hold the ball?" And I really wanted to prove to them that I could.

I was motivated, and I felt like if I dialed it back too much, I'd be giving in. But I definitely made it a balance. The clinical team was a little nervous at first, but I was doing fine through treatment. I felt really strong most of the time. Part of it was, I was young. It probably would have hit me harder if I were seventy-five, or even fifty.

But it was strange: Colleagues wouldn't recognize me in the hallway. Because I looked like a patient, you know? There was that kind of oddity, like, "OK, here I am and now I'm on the [examining] table instead of on the tumor board with you discussing things professionally."

■

For me coming to work was almost in a weird way an escape from my own situation, although ironically, I was looking at breast cancer all day.

■

During her treatment, Kimberly created her own circle of "gurus" to help out with different aspects of the breast cancer battle.

You can say you don't want any help, or you can communicate a lot. For me, I assigned "gurus" to do different things for me because they all want to help. If you have a good network of people around you, they want to help you in some way and not just be crying on the phone. And it's nice to let them. For them and you.

You have to be a little Type A about that if you want to coordinate everybody. Or you can assign somebody else to do that. As long as it's not burdening one person a ton, I think it can be really nice to have sort of shared help in lots of different ways, emotionally and physically.

When people would ask "How can I help out," I would respond, "Hey, will you be my guru making music for me to listen to when I'm having infusions? Or help me with finding good recipes when I don't feel like eating much? And help me shop for a wig or headscarf?" And some of them didn't even live near me. It just mentally kind of helped everybody feel like they were on a team, and it felt good to me too.

In some ways, the cancer treatment also drew her closer to her husband. But after her battle, they divorced. (Kimberly is now happily remarried.)

He'd opened a restaurant right before I was diagnosed, and he was really busy with that [but] super supportive. He'd come to all my chemotherapy sessions, and it was actually great quality time for us, in that sense. We'd have to slow down and spend six hours together sitting next to each other, not doing something else. That was true, not just for my marriage, but also for my kids. I was around more. And I had family flying in to help out with the kids every other week or so, so I saw my mom more often and my husband's mom.

But I think it was a scary thing for my husband. He would stay late at work sometimes. We would have our day together during chemotherapy, and then he'd kind of disappear and do all the stuff he had to do. He ended up having a midlife crisis a few years down the line. How much it had to do with [the cancer], I don't know.

THE COMEBACK

As for Kimberly, she has stayed the path professionally, doing research into guidelines for HER2-positive cancer and channeling her struggle into *Red Sunshine: A Story of Strength and Inspiration from a Doctor Who Survived Stage 3 Breast Cancer*, published in 2011. Her experience also brought a different dimension to the training of the department's residents. None of them had much direct interaction with patients and survivors in their practice, but now they work alongside one.

> I had only finished residency a few years before, so I was a similar age to some of them, and they were learning how to diagnose cancer. But we don't interact with patients all the time, so we're not constantly seeing what they're going through. I think [my breast cancer experience] had a big impact on them, and on my department in general. [It makes you think], "Oh, this is the reality that this can happen to any of us, and what we do is important because patients depend on us for accurately diagnosing them."

GEETA RAO GUPTA

I always felt I was empathetic to the women I was
working for, but that level of empathy goes up 100 percent [when you have breast cancer].

■ ■ ■

For over a decade, Geeta Rao Gupta served as the president of the International Centre for Research on Women (ICRW), a non-profit based in Washington, D.C., dedicated to using research to shape international development policies and programs to empower women and girls. From 2010 to 2011, she was a senior fellow at the Bill and Melinda Gates Foundation, and from 2011 to 2016 she was Deputy Executive Director at UNICEF. Currently, Geeta is the Executive Director of the 3D Program for Girls and Women and Senior Fellow at the United Nations Foundation.

THE DIAGNOSIS

Geeta credits two very special women with saving her life: her sister and her assistant.

Her sister, who was also diagnosed with breast cancer, spoke to her with the bluntness and candor that only a blood relation can really do, keeping her accountable even after Geeta thought she was done with her breast health due diligence.

Her assistant went above and beyond the tasks she was paid to do in order to keep her boss on track with her health, committing some well-meaning subterfuge so that Geeta was always putting her own care first—even when she didn't know it.

Geeta's other loved ones—her husband and her daughter, as well as her father—made up the rest of her superstar support team. But it was those two women who made the biggest difference in her detecting her cancer in 2006.

My canary in the coal mine was my sister. I had actually scheduled a mammogram that year, in '06, and my sister called to say that she had been for her test, they found a small lump, and it was very tiny but very cancerous. In the course of the conversation she asked, "Have you scheduled your mammogram?" And I said, "Yes, it's coming up." And she said, "Have you done a clinical self-exam?" And I said, "Actually I haven't in a while." So that night, lying in bed, I did an exam and found this big lump. And it was big!

I said to my husband [Arvind], "Oh God, there's something here." He said, "I'm sure it will be benign." I had a history of benign fibroids in my breasts. And I said, "But this one's huge." And so I went for my mammogram.

Then I waited, biting my nails, and my sister, too. I was so anxious. She was on the West Coast, I was in Washington, D.C. It wasn't even that they'd found a lump and it was benign; they didn't find anything.

So I just said, "Phew, clear mammogram," and forgot about it. But then my sister called and she asked, "What did the mammogram say?" And I said, "Clear." She said, "What do you mean 'clear'? Do you have a lump?" I said, "Yes, I felt a lump."

"So feel now, do you feel it?" she asked. I said yes. She said, "Did you tell them you had a lump?" I said, "No, I didn't tell them; I'd hoped they'd find it." My sister told me, "You should go see a doctor."

And then there was another coincidence. My executive assistant at that time, who was a wonderful woman, came into my office a few days later. Something had happened at work that was upsetting me, and I got teary. And she said, "You never cry at work. What's going on?" And I said, "I don't know. That's actually odd." And then I said, "Perhaps I'm anxious a little bit because I have this lump, but the mammogram was clear, and my sister said I should be worried, and I have no time to see a doctor, I'm so busy."

My assistant didn't say anything to me. She called my private physician, because she used to set my doctors' appointments. She told my physician that my sister had been diagnosed with cancer, and that I had a lump. And that physician said, "She shouldn't see me. She should go straight to an oncologist if her sister's got cancer." And so my assistant found out who to see, she got all the details. She made that appointment. That oncologist said to her, "[Geeta] needs to bring her mammogram slides." There was no way my assistant could have gotten [those] on her own, but she called the mammogram clinic that I went to, and they told her she needed an authorization letter to pick them up.

I used to sign, almost on a daily basis, about twenty to thirty thank-you notes to donors to my organization. My assistant didn't mean to fool me. She put the authorization letter in the bottom of that pile. And I just signed it; I didn't read it.

She was surprised I didn't ask anything, but she took the letter, went to the mammogram clinic, picked up my slides, put them in an envelope, put a date appointment on my calendar, and marked it, "Doctor's appointment." So that day I went to the calendar, saw the appointment, and asked if I was supposed to see my personal physician. She said, "No, you have to go to another clinic. And this is the address."

So I jumped into a cab twenty minutes before the appointment. I arrive, and the sign outside the building says "Washington Cancer Center." My heart sank. I called [my assistant] and I said, "Where did you send me?" She said, "Your doctor just said that he's the expert. He'll be the one to tell you." That's how it began.

The week after I went to see the oncologist, I was supposed to leave for London to chair the first meeting on cervical cancer in the developing world, hosted by Merck, at the London School of Hygiene and Tropical Medicine.[22] And I couldn't take that trip, because the oncologist who examined me said, "You're not going anywhere. You're having an ultrasound and then a needle biopsy."

He told me that it was cancerous. I was alone. I hadn't even bothered my husband that day because we had convinced ourselves it would be benign. Obviously, I was shocked, I was crying. I called my husband, and he came rushing over.

I later learned that my breasts are apparently very lumpy and difficult to read on a mammogram. My doctor showed me the mammogram image. He said that once he felt the lump, he could see where it was. But if he hadn't clinically examined me, he may have missed it, too. I no longer have just mammograms. I always have an MRI, too. My insurance hates it, but they are forced to cover it.

My lump was really big. If I remember it, it was 5 centimeters. My sister's lump was .5 millimeters. And mine was deep in my breast. It wasn't on the surface; it was close to my ribcage. The doctors were nervous about metastasis to the bone and to the ribcage. Plus, it was so big that they couldn't do surgery right away because they would have destroyed the architecture of the breast, which would have required a mastectomy.

Geeta had a hard time telling her family about the diagnosis.

The most difficult part of the entire experience was telling people you care for and you love that you are a cause of anxiety to them. That was the worst. Telling my elderly father [Srini Rao, who passed away in 2014], telling my husband, telling my daughter—it was devastating.

My mom had died just two years before, in July 2004. My diagnosis was in December 2006. My father had gone back to India for the first time since my mother's death, in August 2006. He had been gone for three months, and I got the news while he was away. So to tell him over the phone was horrible, as one who just experienced a loss—and this news from both of his daughters.

I think I told him about both of us, and then my sister called him. Because I'm the older sister and he lived with us. I remember telling him he should finish out his time in India and then come, there's no hurry. And he said, "No, I'm getting on the next plane. I'm coming home." In my house, the couch in the family room downstairs was where I used to lie down after my chemo, most days. And he had his armchair right in front of me, so he would keep watch on me, very sweetly. He was a dear, dear man. So telling him was devastating.

My daughter Nayna was in college at Northwestern. I was diagnosed about eight months before she graduated. She came back on a school break. I didn't tell her while she was away because she was coming back in another week, so I thought, "What's the point?"

I remember picking her up at the airport, driving home, not telling her, and then waiting, thinking, "When's the right time to tell her?" And she, being a normal college kid, coming home to where she grew up, immediately contacted all her friends because everybody was home on vacation. Then all of a sudden the doorbell rang, and there were all of her girlfriends. And I thought, "Now, when do I tell her?" Because her girlfriends were all downstairs, and she was in the bathroom getting ready to go down to greet them. I just thought I should tell her before she sees them all, so she can get their support. And I remember opening the door and saying to her, "I need to talk to you." Her dad and I told her the news, and her first reaction was, "Why didn't you tell me right away?" And I said, "Because you were away." Then she banged the door of the bathroom and sat in there for who knows how long.

So I went downstairs and told her friends, "She's getting ready."

Then she walked out of the bathroom, and she just ignored us. She couldn't cope. But it was a good thing I told her then because she did tell her girlfriends. They were able to talk it through. So by the time they left, she was able to come lie down with me and apologize to me for being angry. She just felt out of control and fearful, and I understood because it wasn't just her mother who had cancer, but also her aunt, who she loved.

The most immediate impact was that she didn't want to go back to college. She had the last semester left, and she just fought with us. "I'm going to stay. I want to be with my mom, be here through your treatment." And just the thought of her delaying her graduation because of my illness—nothing could have been worse. So I kept telling her, "It's going to be fine, I'm going to be fine," and then finally she agreed, reluctantly. We took her to the airport. I'll never forget, we were having a cup of coffee before she got onto the plane, and she just said, "I'm not going, and you can't push me to go. I'm not getting on the flight. That's it." And she just sat there. And I just started crying. I said, "I do not want you to delay graduation because of me, and you have to understand my perspective."

And my husband, being the smart man he was, said, "You know what honey? Any time you want to see your mom, I'll buy your ticket. Whatever seat is available, however I can bring you, I'll bring you. So the minute you're sitting in your college and you feel, 'I want to see my mom,' I'll get you on a flight that night." And she came three times. My husband spent whatever it cost. But I feel the guilt that her last semester grades would have been better if it weren't for me. Because it traveled with her, even though I was far away. But she's done fine, so it didn't matter in the long run.

Because she was also so close with her staff at ICRW, it was a similarly emotional experience breaking the news to them.

I first told my senior VP. I said that the doctor had advised me that I could work through it, and that I would like to. And she said, "That's fine, but then you need to inform the office." My doctor's office had a nurse practitioner who had told me that some women like to keep it private, don't talk about it, and just manage their work that way with very few people knowing. And I'm just not that type. I just wanted to tell the world. I know I need support, and it's easier to get it when people know.

So I called my two other VPs, one in charge of programs, one in charge of administration, and told them. Both cried, which was difficult to watch.

Then we talked about how to plan the work, who would take over what if I didn't show. I told them about the chemo. I knew that the third day after chemo, you probably feel down and not well enough to come to work, and then two days later you feel fine, and just when you're absolutely fine it's time for the next chemo. They just decided to play it by ear. I told the rest of the team in a staff meeting, "I'm going to be fine, but this is how it's going to be for the next few years."

THE BATTLE

Geeta received neoadjuvant chemotherapy, followed by a lumpectomy.

I had the chemo every two weeks. They hoped the chemo would [reduce] the size of the lump so that they wouldn't have to take out that much tissue when they went into surgery. But, in fact, that did not happen. The chemo had no effect on the size of the lump. It was very scary.

Because the lump didn't decrease, I had to have a plastic surgeon work on both breasts. I'm a public speaker, and they said if they removed that much from the right breast, which had the cancer, it would drop. Even if they pulled the muscle up to hold my breast up, it would be much smaller than the left, and I said, "No, I couldn't let that happen because it would be publicly visible." So they had to do a breast reduction on the left to match the right one.

That was also very funny. When I went to see the plastic surgeon, he was hysterical. Everybody in the waiting room was clearly a woman who wanted to look beautiful. And then I was the breast cancer patient, here only for the purpose of getting rid of an illness. My oncologist had recommended him because he's an exceptional plastic surgeon. I remember, my husband was in the room with me, and the surgeon looked at my breasts and said, "While we're in there, would you like me to lift them?" and he was giving me all these suggestions. And I said, "Time out! Literally, time out. I'm only here for one reason: to get rid of my cancer and for me to be normal enough to face a crowd. That's it. Nothing else."

He went on, and on, and on: "No, but it's simple enough to do, and I could take off some fat from here and some fat from there, and it would be paid for by insurance." I said no. And my husband still laughs about it, because I said, "My breasts have served me very well. They've served my husband well. They served my baby well. They served me well. I don't need anything more to be done to them."

Another seemingly cosmetic problem cut further than skin-deep: the loss of her hair.

It was a reminder on a daily basis that you're sick. Secondly, nobody had told me: It actually hurts to lose your hair! Everybody advised me, "Just shave your hair off when you start chemo." And I was this hopeful creature. I thought, "Maybe I won't lose it all. Maybe I'll keep it." So I didn't get it shaved off. And I cannot tell you how painful it was, because the chemotherapy works at the pore, at the root of the hair. It kills the root. You know how sometimes when you have a part in your hair, and when you sleep awkwardly it goes against the part? You know how it hurts? Every single pore, if you can imagine, felt that way, as if somebody had moved it the wrong way.

It hurt so badly when you put your head down on the pillow. It would feel like pins and needles. The other thing is the way your hair falls: It falls in tufts, which they said would be traumatic. That's why they say just shave it off. And I kept saying no, and then finally I just called my hairdresser to my home.

I think I wore a wig the first week because I had gotten the wig in advance, but I didn't like it, so I switched to a turban. People were very careful about what they said. Some people get so nervous they would say the wrong thing. And then other people are so caring and ask you every day, "How are you doing today, and how is it going today, and how did that last treatment go?"

And then there are still others who immediately process it as, "Can I get breast cancer?" Which is a very self-protective kind of mechanism. And so their questioning was all about, "Where did you live? Was it some place that's toxic? Was it some kind of food you ate?" Which for me was jarring, because it was like blaming the victim. I didn't do anything wrong, I promise you!

Immediately, then you start thinking, "Did I not exercise enough? Maybe I need a less strenuous job." It's crazy-making, because you have no history and then suddenly you and your sister both have cancer.

■

I said, "My breasts have served me very well. They've served my husband well. They served my baby well. They served me well. I don't need anything more to be done to them."

■

The chemotherapy also gave Geeta bad mouth sores.

There were holes in my tongue, it was horrible. You don't feel like eating, and then when you want to eat, everything would burn. One [taste] is metallic because of the chemo [affecting] your taste buds. But this used to actually burn. They give you what they call "magic mouthwash," which numbs it all. It's like going to the dentist—it's completely numb inside, but then you can't taste a thing. So I would avoid using that, and I couldn't eat. So my father would get very upset. Indian dads, you know.

Despite her discomfort, Geeta was lucky to have such an amazing support system.

Arvind was a total rock. He wasn't being overly conciliatory or overly caring. He was just himself. But understanding. I remember an occasion where were planning to go out to dinner with friends, and that particular day I was just feeling very self-pitying. I was just in one of those moods, thinking, "Why did this happen to me, why didn't it happen to anybody else?" And I said, "I don't want to go for the dinner. I don't feel like it." Also, your skin complexion changes—you feel sallow and ugly—and I had some acne that I didn't use to have. And he said, "That's fine, we won't go." And I said, "Why don't you? You can go." And he said, "You know what? It's a good idea. Yeah, I'll go. It'll help me and it'll help you." He was very pragmatic about things like that. He was also very good with my father in just keeping the routine going, because my dad was elderly and needed his meals on time.

My colleagues from the outset were incredibly supportive. Many offered to help. When I was thinking where I should get treatment, someone said Sloan Kettering in New York is the place. I remember saying, "I don't have a place to stay there, how would that work?" And how many people came out of the woodwork offering me their apartment! So people were very, very supportive. I had, in that sense, an extremely positive experience.

[Work] helped me feel a sense of normalcy, for certain. But lucky for me, I was the head of the institution, so I could call the shots a little bit. And I had a board that was incredibly supportive. So it was the easiest thing for me. I've since heard of women who are professors who didn't tell anybody or who are at corporations where it'll affect your career growth—there was none of that for me. So there were no negative downsides that I could see at the time.

A lot of women have explained to me that they felt like a lame duck—kept out of things and not involved in decisions. My office didn't treat it that way, somehow. I was very involved. I remember we used to do these annual galas to fundraise. And we had one when I was in the middle of chemo, and the office did a lot of the work behind it, but I was still involved in the decision-making around it and the planning around it.

■

Immediately, then you start thinking, "Did I not

exercise enough? Maybe I need a less strenuous job."

It's crazy-making, because you have no history and

then suddenly you and your sister both have cancer.

■

The gala was a way for Geeta to show that she was still the same viva-cious woman she was before she was diagnosed with cancer.

I love music and I love to dance. So we always had a band at the end of the galas I planned. I remember, during that particular gala when I was sick, I was determined to dance to show the office that I was fine. And then once I started dancing, I couldn't stop. And it was in the middle of my chemo treatment. I had arrived late, I'd been sitting most of the time, but when the music started, I just thought, "You know what, I just should dance because it's going to get everybody in gear." And it was wonderful. And a lot of my staff afterwards said that it was a joy to see.

Meryl Streep was actually my guest for that gala, and she gave me lots of tips. She had said that someone close to her had had breast cancer, that she knew the person with the perfect wigs. She said, "You just send me a note, and I'll tell you who my wig maker is, and that's the one you should go after." It was somebody who made wigs for her films.

THE COMEBACK
Geeta was already very much in sync with the mission of the organiza-tion she led, but her breast cancer journey made her even more so.

IRCW does research, usually in collaboration with people in the coun-tries in which we are working. The findings should inform policies or pro-grams. I always looked at the user side of health issues and what women need, the gendered angle—because of gender, what obstacles women face in accessing care.

I always felt I was empathetic to the women I was working for, but that level of empathy [went] up 100 percent. The seriousness of the issues for individuals, rather than as statistics, became clearer to me. The challenges of dealing with the health care system unless people are kind and treat you well, how much can go wrong—all that, you become much more profoundly aware of.

It also opened her eyes even more to the sorts of health care challenges women in *this* country face on a regular basis.

I felt very blessed because my insurance covered everything. There's one particular shot which builds up your white blood cell count and red blood cell count, so you're not prone to infections. But when I was going through treatment you had to have the shot after every treatment, about two days later. That one shot, if I remember right, was something as enormous as $5,000 each. So when I walked into the doctor's clinic, each time they would then order it from the stockroom, because nobody was allowed to keep a spare one. It had to be signed off by the doctor on the spot.

The thought that those kinds of expensive treatments were available to me and allowed me to maintain as much normalcy in my day-to-day living as possible, and were not available to women in poorer countries, or even in this country, was really an eye-opener for me. I remember one day sitting in the waiting room to see my doctor, and there was a woman negotiating with her insurance company at the reception desk, trying to convince them, "No, it's OK, I've not been fired, I'm just on leave." But she had been fired, and there was no insurance to finish her chemo. Can you imagine? I remember crying, sitting in that room. And I remember the receptionist was devastated because she had to tell her, "Ma'am, there's nothing we can do." You can continue if you can pay, but there was no way she could afford it.

Once her treatment was all finished, Geeta also experienced the fear (which many breast cancer patients face), not just of a recurrence, but of the worry that, now that you're not in treatment all the time, something bad might happen.

> You've been through this, they tell you you're OK, and then the fear sets in. And that fear lasts a long time. It's like the sword hanging over your head, that you're now a breast cancer patient. I remember the worst, most terrible incident ever I had was maybe two or three months after it was all over. I went in for a checkup and mentioned I used to have breast cancer, and there was a nurse standing there who said, "Lady, once a breast cancer patient, always a breast cancer patient." I'll never forget it. I wanted to smack her face.
>
> But in retrospect, when I think about it, it was absolutely the wrong thing for her to say, but it's the truth. I've had many episodes over the years of, "We've seen something." Once you've had breast cancer and they see even the most minor thing, they explore it to the nth degree. They won't say anything, but they have you do an ultrasound, an MRI, a needle biopsy, then, "We'll let you know." So I've been through that at least three times in the ten years [since]. That fear is horrible.
>
> Most of [the breast cancer experience], I've forgotten, frankly. Some things I haven't forgotten: bone pain, head pain, the sores. But everything else—the tiredness, the fatigue—I don't remember that much.

Geeta did experience a few side effects after her treatment. She recalls an episode where her post-chemotherapy shots made her bones ache so much that she collapsed in a store. She also now has atrial fibrillation—a condition that causes an irregular, sped-up heartbeat—as a result of her radiation. But overall, she's doing well and is grateful for the lessons breast cancer taught her.

> I remember someone saying that cancer's given them a perspective on life, and that they no longer are going to be in the rat race that they've been in, and they're now going to change jobs.
>
> Both my sister and I felt that we were doing exactly what we wanted to do. We never wanted to change what we were doing, and that this certainly wasn't going to do it. It didn't give me the kind of perspective of

"I should do something different." It gave me the perspective that I was doing exactly the right thing—and now more than ever.

ELLEN NOGHÈS & SALLY OREN
ON CREATING A CANCER SISTERHOOD

Ellen Noghès is a four-time cancer survivor, cancer prevention advocate, and wife of former Monegasque ambassador Gilles Noghès. She was born and raised in Michigan and met Gilles while working in France.

Sally Oren sits on the US advisory council of IsraAID, an Israel-based international NGO, where she began volunteering in 2012 as a goodwill ambassador. She also served as the president of the board of Hadassah International Israel, a Jewish women's organization, and was previously married to former Israeli ambassador Michael Oren. Sally grew up in San Francisco, California.

Against their will, they both joined an exclusive club that is surprisingly large: ambassadors, and ambassadorial spouses, who have battled breast cancer far from home. And together, they used their own experiences to make it easier for those who came after them.

Ellen: I was first diagnosed with breast cancer in 2001. In all, I've had three battles with melanoma, and four diagnoses of cancer in total. My husband was #2 at the Monegasque embassy in Paris, and it was January of my fiftieth year. My birthday was in December, and I went for a regular mammogram. They found something at the American hospital in Paris that was suspicious, and I just remember sitting in that office that day, having this French doctor tell me I had breast cancer. I've always said that breast cancer speak is a foreign language anyway. And to receive the diagnosis in French was just shocking to me. But the most important part of that whole story was, we were very involved with the diplomatic community in Paris and we were very good friends with the ambassador of Cyprus and his wife, Calliope, who we called Popi. We would see each other at these diplomatic events, and we'd go out to dinner, and we never, ever mentioned [breast cancer].

The Cypriot ambassador moved on to Ireland, and we moved on to Switzerland, and then we found ourselves in 2004 in New York for the United Nations, together. And there was this women's club in New York that wanted to have diplomatic members, so they had invited both the wife of Cyprus and myself to become members. We had to write our little bios that they would put in the program. I said, "Oh, I don't know what to write. Send me, Popi, what you wrote." And in her little bio, she wrote that she was a breast cancer survivor. She was ten years younger than me at the time—forty-three. So I called her up, and I said, "Calliope, when did you have breast cancer?" "Oh, in Paris!" she said. And I said, "But when?" And she said, "January, February 2001." That's when I was diagnosed. And I said, "Oh my God, Calliope, so was I. We were seeing one another at these diplomatic events, and we weren't sharing that!"

Ellen thought about all the missed opportunities for the two of them to commiserate. She had had her husband to support her during her treatment, and a healthy social life, but she had endured the rigors of her treatment without someone to relate to.

Ellen: It was challenging. Part of it was, despite the fact I was being treated at the American hospital in Paris, they didn't have a coordinated treatment system set up. Nowadays, at least here in the United States, you have comprehensive care. They're not leaving you to just see your surgeon and go back home. There's people looking out for you.

My doctors told me that for the radiation, I needed cotton bras, for example. I went out looking in Paris, in the Galeries Lafayette. They didn't have cotton bras. I didn't know where to find cotton underwear that would feel comfortable if my skin got burned by the radiation. And I didn't know anyone who had had breast cancer! I didn't have anyone to talk to, and I was away from friends and family. Even in the United States I didn't have friends who were calling me and saying, "I've been through this."

And so, one night in my deep sleep, I just sat up in New York in the middle of the night and said, "Oh my God, there is a moral to our story! You need to talk about it. If Popi and I had talked about it, we could have had lunch together after radiation treatment. We could have found support. Our husbands would have felt more comfortable." But we never mentioned it! And we found out three years later we were going through the same thing at the same time. So that was my driving force, in New York, to say, "We've got to take this story and make sure everyone knows you've got to talk about it!"

We decided to have a joint reception at home and invite the wives of all the ambassadors of the United Nations. And seventy-five women came from six of the seven continents. I was introduced to my oncologist in New York through Calliope, so she came to speak at our residence. We called it the "Pink Party," and we decorated everything in pink. Everyone wore a little bit of pink. It just so happened that Prince Albert of Monaco was in town at that time, and I wrote and told him that I was doing this in the name of breast cancer advocacy, and would he grace my party with his presence? He came, and he wore a pink tie. We scheduled two and a half hours for this reception, but it could have gone on much, much longer.

When I got to New York and then Washington, I realized how many women were going through this in a foreign country, getting diagnosed in a foreign language and having health insurance issues. I didn't have health insurance issues in France because my husband was from Monaco, but I know a number of women who struggled with health insurance because of cash flow and payments and chemo treatments that cost so much. And you just think, you really don't need that when your focus and your energy should be just going to keeping a smile on your face and staying strong and staying positive.

So after Prince Albert tasked Gilles with setting up the first embassy of Monaco in Washington, Ellen was determined to continue her outreach, convinced that there were members of the diplomatic community who would appreciate her help.

> *Ellen: One of our neighbors in Washington was the ambassador of Afghanistan. I'd be out walking my dogs and we'd see them, and then I was invited to join one of the women's groups in Washington [known as International Clubs, open to spouses of ambassadors, members of Congress, Supreme Court justices, etc.]. The wife of the Afghan ambassador was also in my club, and I found out she was diagnosed with breast cancer. I called her and told her to come over. We talked. And then after Afghanistan, it was Slovenia; after Slovenia, it was Norway; after Norway, we discovered Sally, and it just turned into this club. We certainly didn't want to grow, but it grew! So we just started this informal group, and we'd take turns hosting. It became like soul sisters.*

This was exactly the sort of group that Sally Oren, the newly arrived wife of Israeli ambassador Michael Oren, needed. She had had her own experience where her breast cancer life collided with her diplomatic life.

> *Sally: When I was diagnosed in Washington, we had been at the embassy for two years.*
> *One of the things we did at the residence was have gatherings of different communities, and they were always around music. Our first event was with the American-Irish community. There are a couple excellent Israeli Irish bands—Israelis who play Irish music—so we invited one of them, because we always highlighted Israeli musicians.*
> *So the first event happened to be the night before my surgery, the lumpectomy. It was a great distraction for me. We had a blast. We had about seventy guests and there was fabulous music. It was a great evening. And then everybody left, and a*

couple hours later, we piled in the car and drove off to the hospital.

When we were leaving the hospital, when Michael was wheeling me out in a wheelchair, we bumped into the director of the hospital, who had been at our house the night before. And he said, "Why didn't you tell me?!" I wasn't about to tell him because I didn't want to put a damper on the event. I had been having a great time, and it totally took my mind off the fact that I was having surgery.

For support, Sally turned to one of her diplomatic friends who had also been through breast cancer.

Sally: *There was one woman, the wife of the Norwegian ambassador, who I was close to. And she had had breast cancer the year before I did. She told me she's in this support group—a very eclectic group. There were women from Norway, Monaco, Switzerland, Malaysia, Afghanistan—not a group that you would typically think would club together.*

They were great. You can be more intimate with people who are going through the same experience as you. And also, you can be irreverent. You can be funny. Sometimes, people don't know how to behave [around people with breast cancer]. It's hard for them. I don't blame them, but they don't quite know what to do with someone's diagnosis. But we laughed together. There was an ease at being able to express yourself. And you're seeing all these survivors. And that's comforting.

Ellen: *For instance, one evening we were gathered around the island in my kitchen. We wouldn't do this formally. We'd always sit in the kitchen, and I'd serve wine or champagne or water or whatever, but it was like a happy hour. And one of the women had chemo to try to reduce her tumor prior to surgery. So she'd gone through her chemo and she admitted to us that she was scared to death of the surgery. And we were all saying, "Oh my God, that's the easiest part! Don't worry about that." But she kept going, and we all whipped up our tops and shared with* her our scars. So we were all topless in my kitchen, saying, "Look! My surgery was done in Paris, this was done here, this was done there. This is the least of your worries!" We laugh to this day over that evening.

Sally: We all shared our own stories. And everybody's was different. There was uterine cancer, cervical cancer. We also had a woman who became active in the group who never had had cancer, but her daughter had a rare blood disease that is similar to leukemia. And everybody had a different experience. I had a lumpectomy and radiation [for stage I, estrogen receptor-positive breast cancer]. And we discussed the different treatments.

There was one dilemma I had involving a test called oncotyping,* which is done when you've had early-stage breast cancer. They send a sample of the tissue to this lab in L.A. and they give you a recurrence score.** My score was 21, which my doctor considered borderline. But it was scary to be borderline. I was having to consider, "Do I want to have chemo?" It's so dramatic and so extreme. So my doctor decided to get a second opinion, and he said, "If that doctor equivocates, then we can decide together. If he says yes, you should have chemo, I would say you should definitely go for it. And then if he says no, then it's no."

They came back with a pretty resounding "no," which was a huge relief for me, but then, it always leaves questions. Some of these women in my support group had had recurrences of cancer and more than one bout with chemo. And they would tell me, "You made the right decision; it's good you're just having radiation."

And the truth is, we didn't talk about cancer very much. We just had fun. We talked about a lot of other things. We didn't talk about politics, either. Everybody was just very relaxed. The only other thing we would discuss regularly was when people went

---

* A genomic test which can help determine her risk for recurrence and recommended treatment in the event of a recurrence.
** In women older than 50, a score of 26 or above means the benefits of chemotherapy are likely to be greater than the risks of side effects.

for their annual tests, and fireworks would go off when they were clean. That was always wonderful. We were able to celebrate each other's annual or bi-annual test results.

Diplomatic life is exciting, if nothing else, but it also means that physical ties are fleeting. After a while, this core group of women dispersed to all corners of the world for their next assignments. Sally and Michael Oren subsequently divorced, and Sally is back in Israel. Ellen and her husband retired to her native northern Michigan. But all of the women are connected for life.

> ***Sally:*** *We're still in touch with one another, because we had this special bond. A few years ago, the woman who first brought me into the group, whose husband is a minister in Norway, visited Israel so we got together in Jerusalem.*
>
> ***Ellen:*** *Norway went back to Norway, Sally went back to Israel, Slovenia was in The Hague and they're going back to Slovenia, Switzerland's back in Switzerland.*
>
> *We exchange emails and we'll write, "Dear Soul Sisters..." Months can go by. But then we catch up, and someone sends a picture of a grandchild, or someone sends a picture of a full moon, and we all think of one another.*
>
> *We've been retired, living up north in Michigan. I had my mammogram a few years ago and had a scare in my other breast. They had to do a biopsy. I was like, "Oh my God! Don't tell me now that it's the other one." And I shared this with all of them, and from all corners of the world—Israel, Norway, Switzerland—they like held my hand across the ocean all the way through it until I got the report that it was benign.*

DR. MARISA WEISS

My life has been very serious as a breast cancer doctor,
not just in the hospital but around the world through
Breastcancer.org. And then my own life gets caught in
the crossfires. It was very tricky.

■ ■ ■

Dr. Marisa Weiss is a breast oncologist and the founder of Living Beyond
Breast Cancer and Breastcancer.org, two leading resources for breast
cancer survivors. She is also Director of Breast Radiation Oncology and
Breast Health Outreach at Lankenau Medical Center outside of Phila-
delphia, Pennsylvania.

As a breast oncologist, she realized that there were few available resources for patients who had recently finished treatment for early-stage
breast cancer. As many of the women in this book have testified, the fear
of cancer doesn't go away when your chemo, radiation, and/or surgeries
are done. It lingers, and in some cases, can intensify. So in 1991, Marisa
held a conference with the help of some of her patients, talking to them
about what information they'd like to see more of from providers and
establishing a community of survivors to swap stories and advice. That
was the foundation for Living Beyond Breast Cancer, a nonprofit organization that now holds twice-annual conferences and has a Breast Cancer Helpline to help survivors get in touch with volunteers who have
gone through similar experiences.

In 2000, she built on the success of that organization by setting up
Breastcancer.org, a leading patient-focused, online resource that covers
just about any question about breast cancer that a new patient—or any
patient, frankly—might have.

THE DIAGNOSIS

Marisa's leadership, both as a breast cancer doctor and the founder of a web community, had helped countless people well before she was diagnosed herself in 2010, at age fifty-one. She had early-stage breast cancer but prefers not to share specifics.

On a Friday, right after the biopsy and the MRI [that led to the diagnosis], I had to give this keynote presentation to a luncheon full of hundreds of women about breast cancer.

And then Monday, I found out the pathology. I was seeing patients and I came back to my office and the pathologist was sitting in my office, unannounced, and said that it came back breast cancer.

THE BATTLE

Marisa refers to herself as a "dual citizen" of the breast cancer world: both patient and provider, the giver and receiver of medical information and guidance.

I know what's at stake and how it feels to have to be worried about your future, and knowing that all of a sudden, your whole life is hijacked by this diagnosis. And that your life's at risk and it's going to be up to you to rise up and deal with it, and that no one else is going to do it for you.

And the fact is, care is haphazard. I had the best care possible, and there were still major gaps. And I was a breast cancer expert! It's hard to imagine what it's like for somebody who is without that expertise. I understand that even the smartest people, with the best education, have their literacy level plummet when they're diagnosed because they're overwhelmed, anxious, and confused and they just have a rough time making sense of everything.

It's also easy to disappear from the system. For example, you can have a procedure and then disappear. Some doctors may not call you. You might have to call them. It's amazing how busy health care professionals can be, and sometimes it's up to you to keep things moving.

One of the areas that can be delayed is genomic testing, like oncotype [to test a group of genes to see how a cancer is likely to behave].

That's an error that can fall through the cracks. I brought it up in a proactive way. My doctor would have brought it up eventually; I wanted it as soon as possible.

●

I had the best care possible, and there were
still major gaps. And I was a breast cancer expert!
It's hard to imagine what it's like for somebody
who is without that expertise.

●

Marisa was already quite visible in the breast cancer world, and her dual citizenship made her even more so.

My life has been very serious as a breast cancer doctor, not just in the hospital, but around the world through Breastcancer.org. And then my own life gets caught in the crossfires. It was very tricky.

When I was diagnosed there were many millions of women who were dependent on me [through Breastcancer.org]. And I take care of a large number of patients. The people who were dependent on me were freaked out about [whether] I could be available to them. And then a lot of people reacted by saying, "I want to do what she did," or, "I want to know if what I did was the same as what she did," implying that what I did was the right thing, assuming that it would be the "correct" thing to do.

I had to go back to work very quickly, two weeks after my surgery. I was still in a lot of pain, and yet I was responsible for taking care of people's lives. That meant not taking pain medication so I could be fully cognitively present. I only took over-the-counter medicine.

THE COMEBACK

Besides her surgical procedure, which she declined to detail, she went on long-term anti-estrogen therapy and has been more vigilant about weight management, alcohol intake, and physical activity.

> I was learning how to manage, long-term, things that have always been a push-pull in my life. So on a daily basis, that involves making sure I eat a mostly vegetarian-based diet, making sure I got things from organic sources. It creates a high level of vigilance. And I had a lot of different doctors and follow-ups. It just takes over in all kinds of ways. There's not a day that goes by that you don't think about it, and I'm ten years out.

The U.S. Preventive Services Task Force recommends women between the ages of fifty and seventy-four years have screenings every two years.[23] Marisa believes that is way too late and too infrequent, and that, without any other genetic indicators, women should begin getting annual mammograms by age forty.

> Breast cancer is the most common cancer to affect women,[24] and it happens at the prime of life. So it makes sense to minimize your risk and do whatever you can that's reasonable to reduce your risk of breast cancer. That includes prevention, and it also includes early detection. Mammography is the most effective strategy. I'm not saying it's pleasant, but it's relatively easy to do. And it's been proven to help save lives. Until we have better, much more validated methods of determining who needs a mammogram and who doesn't, I recommend sticking to annual mammography starting at age forty for women in general. And if you're a woman at higher risk because of BRCA1 or an inherited genetic mutation, then more frequent surveillance and different techniques besides just mammography are appropriate.

Since its launch in 2000, Breastcancer.org has grown to become a several hundred thousand-strong community of peer-to-peer users—mostly breast cancer survivors and their caretakers—who talk to each other via message boards tailored to different stops on the breast cancer path.

The goal of Breastcancer.org is to help each person get the best care possible, [and to] feel cared for and connected to a community of people who have been there and want to help them get through to the other side. People may not have access to the best information or the best doctors, or even know where to start. We knew we couldn't change the reality of getting that phone call, telling you that [you have] breast cancer. But we can change everything that happens after that moment.

NOTES

1. Thomas, Sandra, Maureen Groer, Mitzi Davis, Patricia Droppleman, Johnie Mozingo, and Margaret Pierce. "Anger and cancer: an analysis of the linkages." *Cancer Nursing* 23, no. 5 (October 2000). https://www.ncbi.nlm.nih.gov/pubmed/11037954.

2. *The Pink Fund.* "New Survey Shows the Increased Financial Burden on Breast Cancer's Youngest Survivors." 2018. www.pinkfund.org/wp-content/uploads/2019/11/TPF_Survey20172018A.pdf.

3. *The Pink Fund.* "Transportation Challenges During Breast Cancer Treatment." October 2019. https://www.pinkfund.org/about/2019survey/.

4. Johnson, Rebecca, Franklin Chien, and Archie Bleyer. "Incidence of Breast Cancer With Distant Involvement Among Women in the United States, 1976 to 2009." *JAMA* 309, no. 8 (2013). https://jamanetwork.com/journals/jama/fullarticle/1656255.

5. *Centers for Disease Control and Prevention.* "Female Breast Cancer and the Environment." National Environment Public Health Tracking. 2016. https://ephtracking.cdc.gov/showCancerBcEnv.action.

6. Powell, Mary. "After Cancer Battle, Feeling Like the 'Luckiest Woman in Vermont.'" *Manchester Journal.* April 14, 2015. https://www.manchesterjournal.com/stories/mary-powell-after-cancer-battle-feeling-like-the-luckiest-woman-in-vermont,55560.

7. Jacobs, Tom. "The burden of the female politician." *The Week.* February 17, 2019. https://theweek.com/articles/820979/burden-female-politician.

8. Canton, Don. *The Bismarck Tribune.* October 12, 2000. https://www.newspapers.com/image/346833991/?terms=heidi%2Bheitkamp%2Bbreast%2Bcancer.

9. Associated Press. *The Bismarck Tribune.* October 30, 2000. https://www.newspapers.com/image/346868969/?terms=heidi%2Bheitkamp%2Bbreast%2Bcancer.

10. Hansel, Jeff. *The Bismarck Tribune.* October 30, 2000. https://www.newspapers.com/image/?clipping_id=38947856&fcfToken=eyJhbGciOiJIUzI1NiIsInR5cCI6IkpX-VCJ9.eyJmcmVlLXZpZXctaWQiOjM0NjgyNjk2NSwiaWF0IjoxNTczNjc2NDMzLC-JleHAiOjE1NzM3NjI4MzN9.SGGj5DwPNadVci1Lwn8_uYkbzJxjwCLtbmIARA5Jx-CQ.

11. *Centers for Disease Control and Prevention.* "Jewish Women and BRCA Gene Mutations." U.S. Department of Health and Human Services. April 5, 2019. https://www.cdc.gov/cancer/breast/young_women/bringyourbrave/hereditary_breast_cancer/jewish_women_brca.htm.

12. *National Cancer Institute.* "BRCA Mutations: Cancer Risk and Genetic Testing: How much does having a *BRCA1* or *BRCA2* gene mutation increase a woman's risk of breast and ovarian cancer?" U.S. Department of Health and Human Services. January 30, 2018. https://www.cancer.gov/about-cancer/causes-prevention/genetics/brca-fact-sheet#how-much-does-having-a-brca1-or-brca2-gene-mutation-increase-a-womans-risk-of-breast-and-ovarian-cancer.

13. Susan G. Komen Organization. "Race and Ethnicity." February 14, 2020. https://ww5.komen.org/BreastCancer/RaceampEthnicity.html.

14. Breastcancer.org. "Do Young Women Have Worst Breast Cancer Outcomes? It Seems to Depend on the Cancer's Characteristics." August 5, 2016. https://www.breastcancer.org/research-news/do-young-women-have-worse-outcomes.

15. *Centers for Disease Control and Prevention.* "Breast Cancer in Young Women." U.S. Department of Health and Human Services. April 5, 2019. https://www.cdc.gov/cancer/breast/young_women/bringyourbrave/breast_cancer_young_women/index.htm.

16. Young Survivor Coalition. "Breast Cancer Statistics in Young Adults." Undated. https://www.youngsurvival.org/learn/about-breast-cancer/statistics#7.

17. Anders, Carey K., David S. Hsu, Gloria Broadwater, Chaitanya R. Acharya, John A. Foekens, Yi ZhangYixin Wang, P. Kelly Marcom, Jeffrey R. Marks, Phillip G. Febbo, Joseph R. Nevins, Anil Potti, and Kimberly L. Blackwell. "Young Age at Diagnosis Correlates With Worse Prognosis and Defines a Subset of Breast Cancers With Shared Patterns of Gene Expression." *Journal of Clinical Oncology.* Presented at the 43rd Annual Meeting of the American Society of Clinical Oncology, Chicago, IL, June 1–5, 2007. https://ascopubs.org/doi/full/10.1200/jco.2007.14.2471?keytype2=tf_ip-secsha&ijkey=fd25ddc2873951492d9332de5cdf4763f714e105&.

18. *Final Update Summary: Breast Cancer: Screening.* U.S. Preventive Services Task Force. February 2018. https://www.uspreventiveservicestaskforce.org/Page/Document/UpdateSummaryFinal/breast-cancer-screening1.

19. Sidney Kimmel Cancer Center. "10 Myths About Breast Cancer." John Hopkins Medicine. https://www.hopkinsmedicine.org/kimmel_cancer_center/centers/breast_cancer_program/treatment_and_services/survivorship/myths.html.

20. Breastcancer.org. "U.S. Breast Cancer Statistics." January 27, 2020. https://www.breastcancer.org/symptoms/understand_bc/statistics.

21. Korkola, James E., Sandy DeVries, Jane Fridlyand, E. Shelley Hwang, Anne L. H. Estep, Yunn-Yi Chen, Karen L. Chew, Shanaz H. Dairkee, Ronald M. Jensen, and Frederic M. Waldman. "Differentiation of Lobular versus Ductal Breast Carcinomas by Expression Microarray Analysis." *Cancer Research* 63, no. 21 (November 2003). https://cancerres.aacrjournals.org/content/63/21/7167.

22. Cervicalcanceraction.org. "Stop Cervical Cancer: Accelerating Global Access to HPV Vaccines Roundtable." Meeting organization by Global Health Strategies, London, England, December 12–13, 2006. http://www.cervicalcanceraction.org/downloads/events/london2006/Stop_Cervical_Cancer_Meeting_Report_FINAL.pdf.

23. *Final Update Summary: Breast Cancer: Screening.* U.S. Preventive Services Task Force. February 2018. https://www.uspreventiveservicestaskforce.org/Page/Document/UpdateSummaryFinal/breast-cancer-screening1.

24. World Cancer Research Fund International. "Worldwide cancer data: Global cancer statistics for the most common cancers." 2018. https://www.wcrf.org/dietandcancer/cancer-trends/worldwide-cancer-data#:~:text=.

RESOURCES

Here are some select resources for anyone who is or knows someone battling breast cancer, or anyone who just wants to be proactive about their breast health. I benefited personally from some of these books and organizations, and I've learned about others through writing this book. Many are suggestions from the wonderful women I interviewed. Of course, this list is far from exhaustive.

BOOKS

If you're interested in learning more about the women profiled in this book, you're in luck: Many of them have written their own books! They are listed below, along with a few of the most popular breast health reference books, plus a few cookbooks and some publications I found to be particularly helpful and insightful.

Allison, Kimberly. *Red Sunshine: A Story of Strength and Inspiration from a Doctor Who Survived Stage 3 Breast Cancer*. Hatherleigh Press, 2011.
    Kimberly's story shows just how difficult an unexpected fight of this kind can be. Her diagnosis came shortly after she became director of breast pathology at Stanford University, yet she felt the same fear of the unknown women from all walks of life feel following a diagnosis.

DioGuardi, Kara. *A Helluva High Note: Surviving Life, Love, and American Idol*. It Books, 2011.
    Kara's book, a beautifully wild, tell-all ride through her life story, predates her cancer diagnosis. And it doesn't shy away from darker times, like her mother's death from ovarian cancer, which led DioGuardi to take the BRCA test years later.

Donaldson, Chris-Tia. *This Is Only a Test: What Breast Cancer Taught Me About Faith, Love, Hair, and Business*. Thank God It's Natural, 2019.
    Chris-Tia tells her amazing story of how she climbed the corporate ladder while also starting up a successful haircare business, the trials and triumphs of being a black woman in corporate America, and how her faith sustained her in her journey through breast cancer.

Field, Valorie Kondos. *Life Is Short, Don't Wait to Dance: Advice and Inspiration from the UCLA Athletics Hall of Fame Coach of 7 NCAA Championship Teams*. Center Street, 2018.
    Valorie explains how she built a legendary gymnastics program without ever having done a tumble or flip herself. Her strategies for finding joy in everything translate into everything she does, whether it's coaching college athletes or facing her breast cancer diagnosis.

Funk, Kristi. *Breasts: The Owner's Manual: Every Woman's Guide to Reducing Cancer Risk, Making Treatment Choices, and Optimizing Outcomes*. Thomas Nelson, 2018.

    Dr. Funk blends science and medicine with humor and common-sense suggestions for how to reduce your risk. She's treated several of the women profiled in this book; reading her book is like stepping into her office for a personal consultation. As she writes: "When you fling excuses and hopelessness at me, I will whack you with a reality check. And when you come to me scared and broken, I will hug you until you're whole again."

Katz, Rebecca. *The Cancer-Fighting Kitchen, Second Edition: Nourishing, Big Flavor Recipes for Cancer Treatment and Recovery*. Ten Speed Press, 2017.

    As soon as you open this book, you already feel like you're doing something good for your body. Katz has an index of ingredients with their specific health benefits, and each recipe is crafted with both flavor and health in mind. This is one of two cookbooks Jennifer Griffin swears by.

Katz, Rebecca. *One Bite at A Time, Revised: Nourishing Recipes for Cancer Survivors and Their Friends*. Celestial Arts, 2008.

    One Bite at a Time is Griffin's other must-buy cookbook for people fighting cancer and their loved ones. This collection of recipes is tailored to people whose taste buds, dietary restrictions, and appetites may all be affected by different types of cancer treatment.

Keshtgar, Mohammed. *The Breast Cancer Cookbook: Over 100 Easy Recipes to Nourish and Boost Health During and After Treatment*. Quadrille Publishing, 2016.

    This book contains very simple, delicious recipes that are applicable for anyone looking to eat healthier, but with particular focus on foods and ingredients that can play a positive role in the prevention and treatment of breast cancer.

Love, Susan. *Dr. Susan Love's Breast Book (Sixth Edition)*. Da Capo Lifelong, 2015.

    This book is alternately referred to as "the Bible for women with breast cancer," and "Breast Cancer 101." It provides all the medical and scientific research a new patient could possibly want, written in accessible language so that you don't have to be an M.D. yourself to understand it. Dr. Love wrote the latest edition, with new information on treatments and methods, after battling leukemia herself, which taught her "a lot about what it feels like to be a patient with no expertise, dependent on a good medical team, family and friends to get you through."

Lucas, Geralyn. *Why I Wore Lipstick: To My Mastectomy*. St. Martin's Griffin, 2005.

    This book is so good, you might want to read it even if you have no connection to breast cancer. Geralyn is a former ABC News producer who writes with a distinct blend of humor and seriousness, never shying away from describing her fears with candor and guiding the reader through every aspect of her own breast cancer battle at just twenty-seven years old.

Lunden, Joan. *Had I Known: A Memoir of Survival*. Harper Paperbacks, 2016.

    Read further about Joan's cancer journey— what it taught her about herself, how it redefined her perception of true beauty, and changed her in unexpected ways—in her own words.

Martin, Shauna. *Daily Greens 4-Day Cleanse: Jump Start Your Health, Reset Your Energy, and Look and Feel Better Than Ever!* Race Point, 2015.

Shauna harnessed the healing powers of food to feel better through chemotherapy. This book dispenses her successful green juice and raw food diet to boost the health of all its readers.

_____. *Energizing Superfood Juices and Smoothies: Nutrient-Dense, Seasonal Recipes to Jump-Start Your Health.* Rock Point, 2019.

Energizing Superfood Juices and Smoothies offers all *Daily Greens 4-Day Cleanse* does and more, including seasonal shopping lists and vegetarian meal recipes.

Queller, Jessica. *Pretty Is What Changes: Impossible Choices, the Breast Cancer Gene, and How I Defied My Destiny.* Spiegel & Grau, 2009.

My plastic surgeon recommended I read this book at the beginning of my journey with the BRCA genetic mutation, the same "breast cancer gene" the author had. I'm so glad I did.

Weiss, Marisa. *Taking Care of Your "Girls": A Breast Health Guide for Girls, Teens and In-Betweens.* Harmony, 2008.

It's never too early to start thinking about breast health. This guide by "dual citizen" Dr. Weiss, both patient and provider, is a great place to start.

ORGANIZATIONS & VIRTUAL COMMUNITIES

Here are some worthy organizations and virtual community websites if you're looking to get involved in breast cancer advocacy or for additional help for you or a loved one. Some of these groups are dedicated to specific communities, and others operate more broadly. Many have peer-to-peer navigation programs which will connect individuals with other group members who have gone through similar experiences in their cancer journey. As always, this list is cultivated through my own experience and reporting, and is far from exhaustive.

Beyond the Shock: https://www.nationalbreastcancer.org/nbcf-programs/beyond-the-shock

In this virtual community hosted by the NBCF, people can browse for answers to questions from medical experts, survivors and patients, and ask their own questions.

BreastCancer.org Community: https://www.breastcancer.org/

This extraordinary collection of forums covers an exponential number of topics, concerns and questions, from "Living Without Reconstruction After a Mastectomy" to sex and relationship matters to members of the LGBTQ community.

Breast Cancer Research Foundation: https://www.bcrf.org/

One of the premiere organizations raising money for breast cancer research worldwide. BCRF has a scientific advisory board, made up of experts in the field, who help guide the investment of each grant dollar.

Bright Pink: https://www.brightpink.org

Founded in 2007 by Lindsay Avner, at the time the youngest woman at 23 to undergo a preventative double-mastectomy, Bright Pink is a national nonprofit organization dedicated to empowering young women to be proactive about their breast and ovarian health.

Facing Our Risk of Cancer Empowered (FORCE): https://www.facingourrisk.org/index.php

FORCE is dedicated to helping individuals and families affected by hereditary breast, ovarian, and related cancers.

Living Beyond Breast Cancer: https://www.lbbc.org/

LBBC has multiple ways to connect to a broader community, including a Breast Cancer Helpline which connects callers and online participants with trained volunteers to support people who are going through breast cancer.

METAvivor: https://www.metavivor.org/

This nonprofit organization exclusively funds research for metastatic breast cancer through a scientific peer-review process.

National Breast Cancer Foundation: https://www.nationalbreastcancer.org/

Founded by breast cancer survivor Janelle Hail in 1991, the NBCF partners with medical facilities to provide free mammograms and diagnostic breast cancer services to underserved women and has numerous resources for breast cancer patients going through treatment and at every stage after that.

Sisters Network: https://www.sistersnetworkinc.org/

Founded in 1994, Sisters Network is the only national African American breast cancer survivorship organization in the United States. Its mission is to save lives and increase attention to the devastating impact that breast cancer has in the African American community.

Sharsheret: https://sharsheret.org/

This national non-profit organization is dedicated to improving the lives of Jewish women and families living with or at increased genetic risk for breast and ovarian cancer. While those are the groups in which Sharsheret specializes, its programs serve all women and men.

Young Survival Coalition: https://www.youngsurvival.org/

The YSC is devoted to helping young adults deal with the unique challenges and needs that young adults affected by breast cancer face.

ACKNOWLEDGMENTS

THIS BOOK WOULD not exist without the generous contributions of all the incredible women—and men—whose stories make up *Beat Breast Cancer Like a Boss*. Many agreed to contribute to this project when it was little more than a pitch on a Google Doc, and I am grateful that they took this project seriously enough to provide their valuable time and candor.

Their managers, assistants, publicists, communications staffs, and partners navigated busy schedules and many time zones to make these interviews a reality. More of them than I'd like to admit graciously rescheduled when breaking news erupted.

Special thanks goes to Steve Roberts, who spoke to me about his beloved late wife, Cokie, and gave me great book-writing advice.

I am also forever indebted to Dr. Lauren Cassell. Ten years after she performed my risk-reducing double mastectomy, she agreed to review my manuscript for medical accuracy. I was amazed at the enthusiasm and vigor she brought to this task. Beyond her technical input, she gave me her perspective as a medical provider. Sometimes we forget that they, too, are human beings, and I am grateful that Dr. Cassell was so thoughtful in explaining how the people in her profession feel about the job they do.

The creation of this book spanned two jobs for me, and I'm grateful to my bosses at both for supporting this passion project: Jonathan Greenberger and Stacia Philips Deshishku at ABC News and Judy Woodruff, Sara Just, and Morgan Till at the *PBS NewsHour*. Martha Raddatz was so supportive from day one (and also connected me with her friend Barbara Delinsky). Howard Schoenholtz cheered me on in this and all other projects I was taking on.

I'm also grateful to my beat colleagues for their patience and indulgence as I talked their ears off about the women I was writing about or when I snuck off for an interview during work hours. That list includes Mary Bruce, Devin Dwyer, Justin Fishel, Mariam Khan, John Parkinson, Emily Schultze, Ben Siegel, Karen Travers, and the mighty foreign team at the *NewsHour*: Morgan, Nick Schifrin, Dan Sagalyn, and Layla Quran.

My agent, Matt Latimer, and Javelin president Keith Urbahn shepherded me through this entire process, from proposal to publication, with great care and skill. Thank you both for being top-notch advocates for your authors.

The team at Diversion Books has made the creation of this book a dream, and I am so grateful to have worked with such a hands-on, enthusiastic group: Publisher Scott Waxman, Executive Editor Keith Wallman, the amazing Melanie Madden, and Emily Hillebrand.

Lastly, my family: my parents, Becky and Max Weinberg, and mother and father-in-law, Sharon and Michael Rogin, all of whom always believed in this project, and my "brilliant, patient, and mischievous" husband, Josh. When asked at our wedding to describe him in three words, those were them, and so they remain. I love you.

INDEX

ABOUT THE AUTHOR

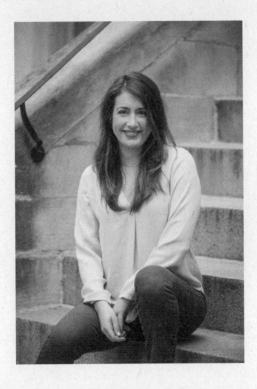

ALI ROGIN IS a producer with the *PBS NewsHour* foreign affairs team, writing and reporting pieces for television and the web. Her reports have also appeared on MSNBC, ABC, SiriusXM, and nationally syndicated FM radio shows. Rogin is a ten-year veteran of D.C.'s political scene, covering the White House, Capitol Hill, and the State Department. She covered the 2012 presidential election, first as a campaign embed during the Republican primary and then as part of the Obama re-election campaign press corps during the general election. During her senior year at New York University, she discovered she had the BRCA1 genetic mutation and decided to have prophylactic surgery before her graduation in 2009. A New Jersey native, Rogin lives with her husband, Josh, and rescue cats, Miles and Dizzy, in Washington, D.C.